A Diary

Through the Lens

We Can Change Lives.....
──我々にできること‥‥──

Nikon   Naoki Hayashi   *Noritake*

はじめに

　私の今日までの人生において、日々のなにげない生活を日記に書き留めるという習慣は一切なかった。そのため文章として、私のこれまでの記録は残されてはいない。しかしながら、私の記憶の中にそれらはさまざまな形として残されている。それは音楽からの追憶であったり、そのときどきの風景であったり、残された香からであったり‥　そして古ぼけた写真からは淡い思い出、せつない記憶が蘇る。

　本書で紹介させていただくいくつかの写真には、私にとって一枚一枚の全てにその時代、その瞬間の背景や行動、そして思い出が鮮烈として刻まれている。もちろん文章で表現されているものではないが、これはまさに私の臨床日記である。

　記録に残された写真からは、時代の流れと共に自分自身が確実に変化してきたことを感じ取ることができる。それは自身の技術の進歩、歯科技工へのより深い理解、そして社会への少しばかりの貢献などである。

　読者の皆様が本書を見る際はわざわざその時間を割くことなく、構えずに楽にして見ていただきたく思う。それは絵本を見るように。そして願わくば、臨床家の皆様が前歯部製作における歯牙形態、ポジション等の決定にある程度自由がきくケースと出会ったとき、本書を気軽に開きその参考にしていただければ幸いに思う。

　最後となるが、多くの歯科医師、歯科技工士、歯科関係者、そして私を周りで支えてくれている人々の貴重な協力なしには、本書を完成することはできなかったであろう。また、このような素晴らしい書籍を製作していただいた、クインテッセンス出版株式会社代表取締役　佐々木一高氏に敬意を表したい。

　われわれは皆良きパートナーであり、最高のチームであることを心から感謝する。

林　直樹

Preface

　I have never been one to keep a diary, and thus I have not written record of my past. However, writing is only one of many forms in which we may document our experiences. The melody of an old song, familiar landscapes and scenery, lingering scents, and old photographs all remind me of past events both happy and bittersweet. Certain photographs, in particular, send me instantly back to the scene, vividly reminding me of my thoughts and actions at that time. Although they are not expressed in writing, such images serve quite effectively as my clinical diary.

　Photography provides evidence of how much I've changed and grown as a dental technician with the times. It documents the improvement of my skills, my deeper understanding of the dental technique, and my modest contributions to society.

　I do not wish you to use your valuable time to read this book, but rather to relax and enjoy it just like you might enjoy going through a child's picture book. I would be happy if you could make use of this book when facing the case of an anterior tooth construction. For example, you might find something in it that can be applied to your understanding of its form and position.

　This book was completed thanks to the united efforts of many dentists, technicians, dentistry related personnel, and others who support me all the time. In addition, I would like to express my appreciation and respect to Quintessence publication corporation chief executive officer Mr. Ikko Sasaki for giving me an opportunity to publish this kind of wonderful book.

　We are all partners, and I am deeply grateful to our team, which is the best one!

序文　　Beauty Through the Lens of the Beholder

レンズは全ての詳細、全ての間違い、全ての要望を先入観なしで見る。
レンズは最高と最低の結果を描写し、我々が感知することのできない自然の力にのみ影響される。
レンズは好みに関係なく真実のみを明らかにする。

　"A Diary -Through the Lens-"では、満足のできる仕事を行ってきた最高のテクニシャンの1人である林直樹氏が描いた、レンズを通してのストーリが語られている。レンズという目を通して氏と私の歯科医療がこのダイアリーに記録されている。私が行っている歯科医療は、最先端を行く材料と磨きぬかれた技術を通して自然を模倣することのできる氏の優れた才能に頼っている。氏の知識の中から引き出され創作された歯科修復物は、機能すると同時に一つのアートでもあり、また氏はそれらを我々の周りの自然の美しさからも学んでいる。

　良好なチームワークをなくしては審美歯科医療の成功は不可能である。治療をするに当たっての機能分析、プレップのデザイン、細かなカスタムシェードが全てのケースにおいて必要とされることは言うまでもない。行うべき治療の全ステップを無計画に取りかかると、十分な満足を得られない平凡な結果に終わってしまう。

　審美歯科は全ての歯科医療の玄関口に位置する様に思う。2005年において"審美的ではない"歯科医療がありえるのだろうか？しかしこの事実は残念なことに、審美治療とは"白いつめ物"で修復治療するべきなのか？補綴物を"周りに調和させる"という目的を持って修復治療するべきか？の区別をつけにくくさせる。どちらも顕在しうるが、区別をするために発言するならば、私は審美歯科医として後者の方を選択したい。氏は今日に見る審美歯科とは何かを、私が明確にするための手助けをしてくれた。機能的な審美修復物とは自然のものとの区別がつかない程のものである。そして審美歯科の世界では、歯科医の目でさえも本物と見間違う審美修復治療が求められている。

　審美歯科医は自然の中にある劣化など全てを含め天然歯に美を見るが、全ての人が天然歯を美しいと見ることはなく、また溝の中の少しのステインや磨耗にも眉をしかめる場合もある。私の情熱は健康的で年相応な範囲で少し若々しい笑顔を作ることにある。どの歯科医も一番難しい審美修復とは単冠の上顎中切歯であるということを知っている。そしてこのタイプの審美修復は歯科医が試みる最も挑戦的な審美改善である。私がこれまで出会ったテクニシャンの中で氏は、隣接歯あるいは口腔内天然歯列全体と補綴物の調和を全ての細部にわたって表現でき、完璧に作成できる唯一のテクニシャンである。

　審美歯科が成功した際、そこから得ることのできる成果は素晴らしいものである。会話や笑顔の中で目立つ見栄えの悪い歯を抱えてきた殆どの患者は、"新しい"歯が過度に白過ぎて目立たないように周りに調和することを要求する。つまり彼らは自然で美しい"普通"の歯を求めている。貧弱な笑顔の人はほとんどの場合、見た目の欠陥にも増してもっと深刻な精神的悩みを抱えている。自身、自己の尊重、最終的には自己の価値にも影響する場合もある。人の笑顔をクリエイトすることは彼らに新しい人生を与えることができる。これこそがまさに審美歯科治療だと私は考えている。

　氏は日々進歩している歯科技術と自然の美を模倣する能力を学ぶことに彼の人生を捧げている。私はそんな林氏と共に仕事ができることをとても光栄に想い止まない。

Dr.Christian W. Hahn
Louisville,Kentucky,USA

Foreword　　Beauty Through the Lens of the Beholder

A lens sees every detail, every fault, and every instance in time without prejudice.
A lens documents our best and worst achievements, influenced only by the intangible forces of nature.
A lens reveals the truth, if you like it or not.

　"A Diary -Through the Lens-" is a story told through the lens of Mr. Naoki Hayashi, one of the finest dental technicians I have had the pleasure to work with. Much my dentistry, with his technical work, is documented in this diary through the critical eye of a lens. My dentistry relies upon his ability and desire to mimic nature to a tee through the use of cutting edge materials and extraordinary skill. He studies the beauty of nature that surrounds us and draws upon this knowledge to create dental restorations that are as much a piece of art as a functional tool. None of this dentistry would have been possible without a great deal of teamwork. Every case required detailed custom shades, preparation design and functional analysis prior to treatment. Jumping into a complicated case without thoroughly planning every step of the procedure will result in mediocre results.

　It seems that cosmetic dentistry is on every dentist's front door. Who is "not" a cosmetic dentist in 2005? This fact unfortunately makes it very difficult to differentiate between "white filling" and truly chameleon type of dentistry. Each has its place, but for the sake of differentiation I am going to refer to the latter as esthetic dentistry. Mr. Hayashi helped me define esthetic dentistry as I see it today: A functional restoration that is indistinguishable from its natural counterparts. Esthetic dentistry seeks to fool even the most experienced eyes—those of a dentist.

　An esthetic dentist sees the beauty in natural dentition, including all the "flaws" that make it real. Not everybody sees natural teeth as beautiful, frowning on grooves, slight stains and abrasions. My passion lies in creating healthy, age-appropriate, yet youthful smiles. Every dentist knows that the most difficult restoration, esthetically, is a single central incisor. This type of restoration is the most challenging cosmetic improvement a dentist can attempt. Mr. Naoki Hayashi is the only technician I have met that truly is able to match every little detail, creating nearly perfect harmony between two adjacent teeth, one being real the other porcelain.

　The rewards of successful esthetic dentistry are great. Most patients, who have lived years with a smile that they were ashamed of, being noticed whenever that speak or laugh, seek to blend in, not stick out with overly white "new" teeth. They desire to look "normal", naturally beautiful. A poor smile is a disability that strikes much deeper than mere cosmetics - it affects confidence, self esteem and ultimately self worth. Restoring someone's smile often gives them a new lease on life. This is what esthetic dentistry is about.

　Mr. Hayashi has dedicated much of his life to the study of advanced dental technology and its ability to mimic the beauty of nature. It has been my pleasure to work with Mr. Naoki Hayashi.

Dr. Christian Hahn
Louisville, Kentucky, USA

序文　　Truly Impressive Natural Art

　真のマスターセラミストアーティスト、林直樹氏と共に仕事ができることはとても光栄なことである。

　1982年以来、ベストで優れた才能を持つ歯科技工士と共に仕事をする機会を永年に渡り探してきた。しかし氏が証明してきたような、質があると同時に芸術性に優れたスキルと情熱を併せ持つ歯科技工士にこれまでめぐり会えることはなかった。治療を行うにあたり、氏の仕事は私の自信を促進してくれるだけに留まらない。それはこの後に続くページで読者の皆さんが目の当たりする通り、我々が行った審美歯科治療前・後の素晴らしい写真を、自信を持って飾ることにより証明されている。

　単純なラミネートベニアの審美修復ケースから、最も困難な前歯1本のみの修復ケースまで、氏は情熱と挑戦する心を研ぎ澄まし、神の手に導かれたかのように患者の口腔内に調和するまで製作し続ける。氏が通常、初回もしくは2回目で正確に色の特色を合わせてくれることは、私にとって何にも変えがたい喜びであり大きな信頼である。患者が氏のオフィスを訪れ、氏自身に直接触れることにより、彼らは氏が自然の美を求めてデンタルアートワークをクリエイトすることに、勤勉かつとても熱心なことに気づき安心を覚える。

　"メディアホワイト"と呼ばれる暗闇の中で真っ白に光り、規則的に並び派手に輝く歯がTVショーメイクオーバーや雑誌等で流行している中、氏のアートは近くで観察を行うと、クラックライン、表面性状や微妙な凹凸が付与されており、更には美しく自然なシェードでキャラクタライズされている。もちろんそれらが驚くほどに口腔内で調和していることは言うまでもない。そしてそれを持った人々は、"素敵な笑顔!"と誰からも絶賛されるであろう。

　氏の所属する"Ultimate Styles Dental Laboratory"と共に仕事をする喜びは、自然で審美的な補綴物をクリエイトする以上のものがある。それは適合性が良く、コンタクト調整の必要もなくマージンの適合は完璧であり、更には長さや形などは私が指示した通りで、なおかつ咬合面の調整も最低限である。私はこのような補綴物をシンプルに口腔内にセットできることに満足感を得ている。そんな我々の日常臨床ケースが本書に多く掲載されている。氏の卓越した技術で歯科材料が使用され、そこから創作された氏の補綴物は本当に印象的である。

　この後に続くページには単に綺麗な歯というだけのものではなく、それ以上の意味を持つ写真も掲載されている。そこに記録されているのは、一般読者が見逃すかもしれない素晴らしい自然の景色である。しかし芸術家たちの眼には、レンズの向こう側にすばらしいストーリーや財産があることを感じ取ることが可能である。"A Diary -Through the Lens-"に目を通した者ならば、氏がまさに天然歯のような審美修復物を製作することで成功の頂点に達していることに留まらず、また素晴らしい写真家でもあるということも一目瞭然である。

　　　　　　　　　　　　　　　　　　　　　　　　　　　　　　　　　　　　　この本を楽しんで下さい。

Dr. Kurt Schneider
Mission Viejo, California, USA

Foreword　　Truly Impressive Natural Art

　It has been such an extreme honor to work with Mr. Naoki Hayashi, a true master ceramic artist. Since 1982, I have sought opportunities to work and learn from the best and brightest talent in dentistry, and no lab technician I've found has come close to the passion, skill, natural artistic ability and overall quality that Mr. Hayashi has demonstrated. Not only has his work enhanced my confidence in treatment planning, but our case acceptance has improved by proudly displaying many of the outstanding before and after photos of our patients that you are about to discover in the following pages.

　From bread and butter multi-veneer treatments to the ultra difficult, single unit anterior crown case, Mr. Hayashi enthusiastically rises to each challenge, ever willing to continue fine tuning his product until it blends harmoniously in the mouth, as if guided by the hand of God. The wonderful thing for me, however, is that he usually nails down the precise matching color characterization on the first or second try. Meeting with our patients in his own office, they often remark how painstakingly precise and passionate he is about the dental artwork created in his pursuit of natural beauty.

　While "media white"—the ultra-white, glow-in-the-dark, straight wall-to-wall brilliance of dental dazzle—is the slick & hip style of modern television makeover shows and magazine articles, Mr. Hayashi's art will "wow" the unsuspecting observer into commenting "Beautiful smile!", with porcelain teeth that when examined closely, look cracked, textured, irregular and characterized with inclusions and beautiful natural shading.

　The joy of working with Mr. Hayashi's Ultimate Styles Laboratory goes beyond creating naturally esthetic dental restorations. I derive satisfaction with the simple delivery of a well fitting, functionally formed restoration where the contacts do not require adjustment, the margins are perfect, the length and proportions are what I prescribed and the occlusion requires only minimal adjustment. Included here are samplings of the typical cases we treat like this every month. With skills that routinely use the most recent advances in restorative materials, Mr. Hayashi's creations are truly impressive.

　The following pages have more than just pretty teeth. Captured here are natural scenes of splendor that the casual observer might overlook, but the artistic eye behind the lens knows there is a story of uniqueness to be shared. Once you have read "A Diary-Through the Lens-", I'm sure you will agree that Mr. Naoki Hayashi has not only achieved the pinnacle of success in re-creating lifelike natural teeth out of porcelain, he's also one heck of a fine photographer!

　　　Enjoy,

Dr. Kurt Schneider
Mission Viejo, California, USA

序文
~ 一つの才能とめぐり合って ~

数年前、一人の若き青年と会う機会があった。その青年は、さまざまな仕事の話しをしていくなかで突然、「青嶋先生、天然歯のようにぬれの良い、つまり吸水性をもった透明ポーセレンの開発はできないでしょうか?」と問うてきた。

この問いに私は非常に驚いた。なぜなら、私も十数年前に同じことを考えていたからだ。"めのう"を観察している時に、硬く、かつ表面が滑沢であるのに吸水性をもっていることに気づいた。しかし、めのうは硬すぎるし熱に脆いので無理としても、他に吸水性をもたせる材料があるのではないかと空想したことがあるからだ。結局は断念せざるをえなかったが、頭の片隅に埋もれていたことが鮮やかに甦ってきた。

私の頭のなかではすでに"ボツ"になっていることだったのだが、この青年、つまり林 直樹氏のことばには、妙なリアリティを感じざるをえず、また歯に対する情熱が頼もしくもあった。

そんな彼が、『A Diary-Through the Lens-』というすばらしい写真集を出版することになった。彼の序文のなかに「記録に残された写真からは、(中略)確実に変化してきたことを感じ取ることができる…」とある。この写真集のどの1枚をとってもすばらしいが、彼にとっては完熟したものではなく、それへの過程なのだ。

この才能ある青年が、さらに幹が太くなり葉を繁らせ、日々にたくさんの実を結び、それが熟していく様を想像するだけで、私の心のなかに新しい血がたぎる。

2005年2月

ペルーラAOSHIMA
青嶋 仁

Foreword
~ Encounter With a Talented Young Man ~

I had a chance to meet a young technician couple of years ago. As I was talking to him about his work, he suddenly asked me, "Do you think it is possible to develop absorbable ceramics that are as translucent and shiny as natural teeth?". His question amazed me because I once had the same idea. When I was looking at agate, I admired its hard and absorbable characteristics, and I noted that even the surface is glossy. However, I decided that it was not a suitable material because it is too hard and easily breaks down by heat. I never did find the material I was searching for, but his question reminded me of my own challenging spirit. I felt a positiveness as well as a great sense of enthusiasm from this young technician, Mr. Naoki Hayashi, and I knew he would do something significant some day.

In this book he publishes a wonderful collection of photographs, entitled "A Diary -Through the Lens-". In the Preface, he says that the photographs are proof that he has "changed and grown." Every photograph in this book is fantastic, and yet he is still on the way to growth. I get very excited when I imagine how this young talented man is growing and accomplishing his dreams.

Hitoshi Aoshima, RDT

はじめに **林 直樹**	•	5
序文／ **Christian W. Hahn**	•	6
序文／ **Kurt R. Schneider**	•	7
序文／ **青嶋 仁**	•	8
光と影—Prologue	•	13
Chapter 1	•	25
Porcelain Fused to Metal Crowns		
Chapter 2	•	41
All Ceramic Crowns		
Chapter 3	•	72
Porcelain Laminate Veneers		
Colors—Epilogue	•	100
術前	•	134
Special Thanks	•	143

CONTENTS

10

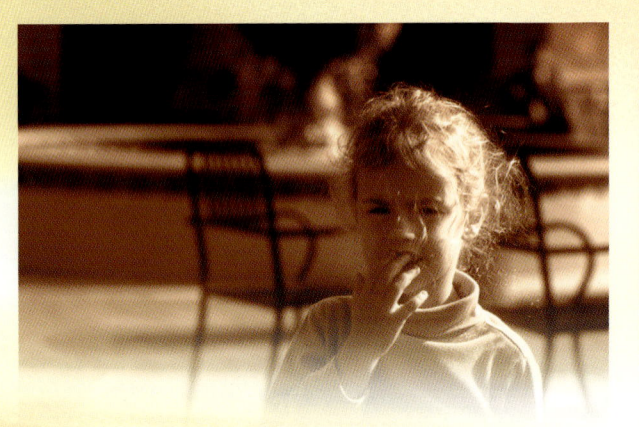

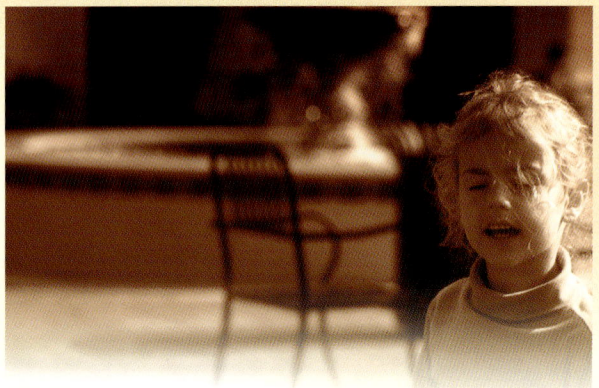

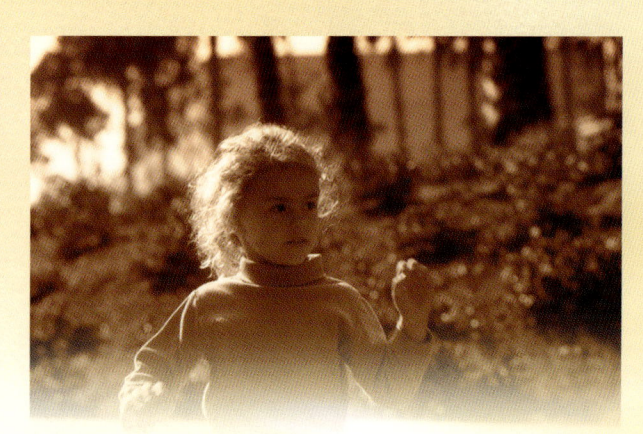

11

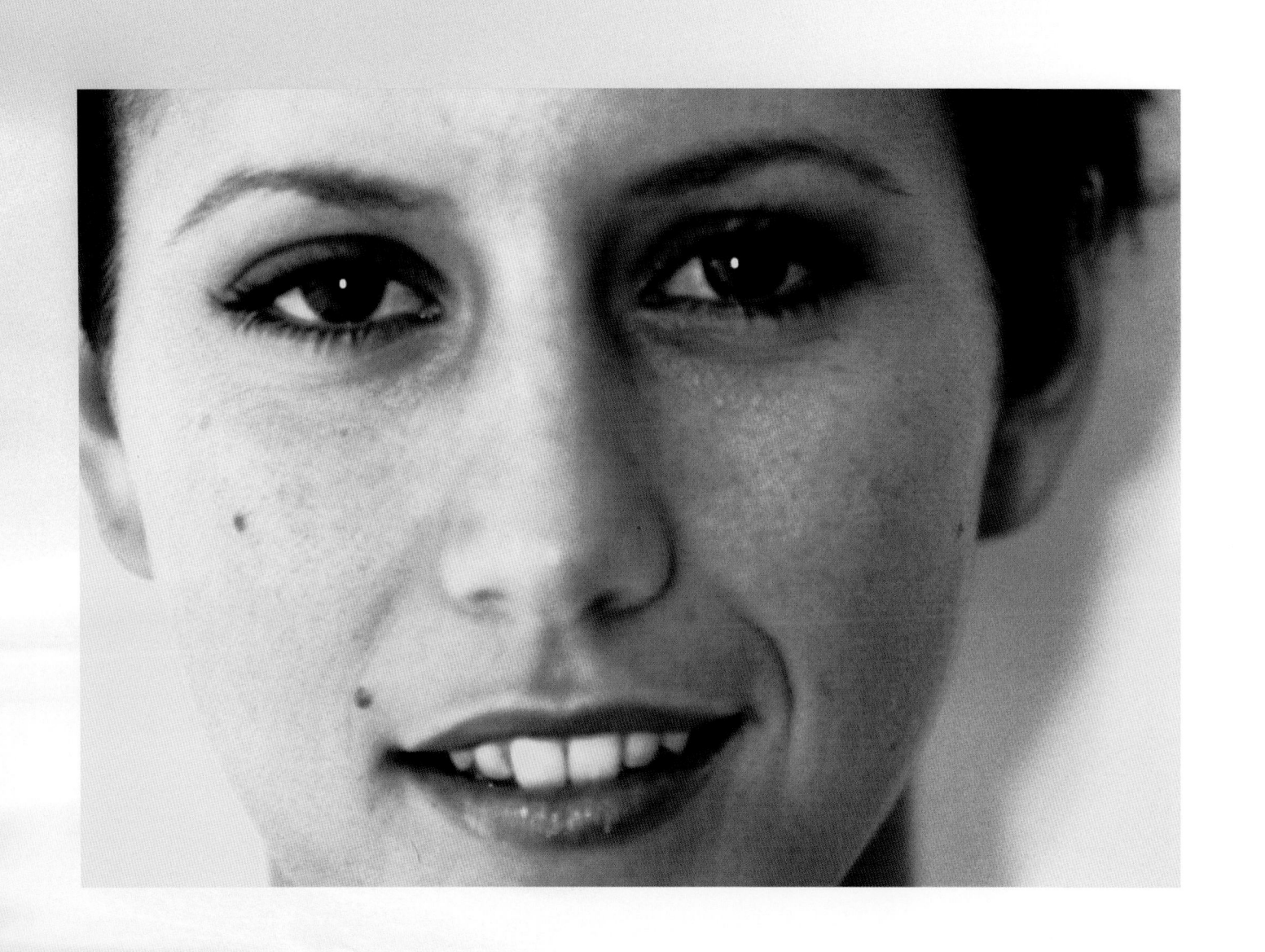

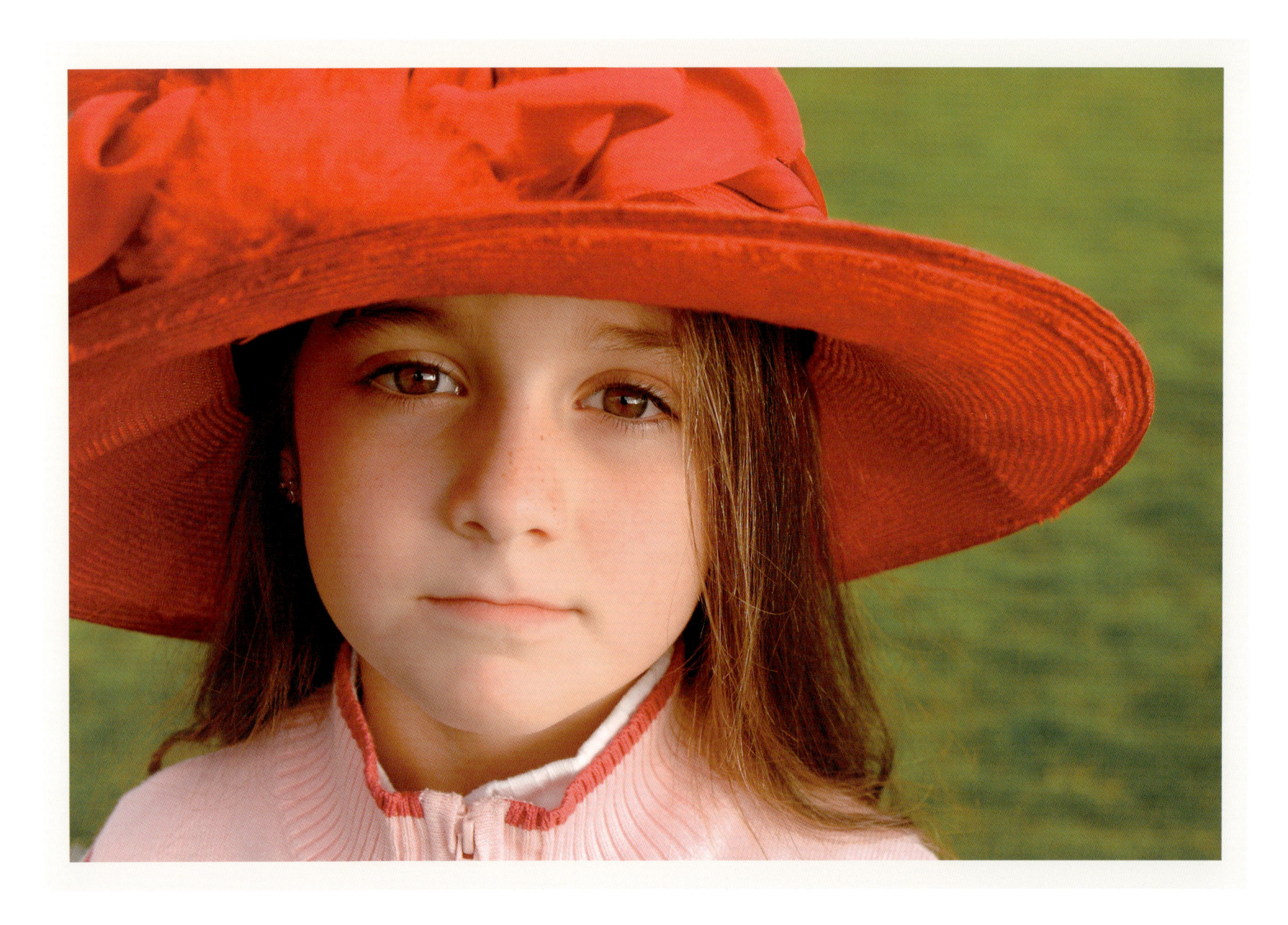

A Diary
Through the Lens

14

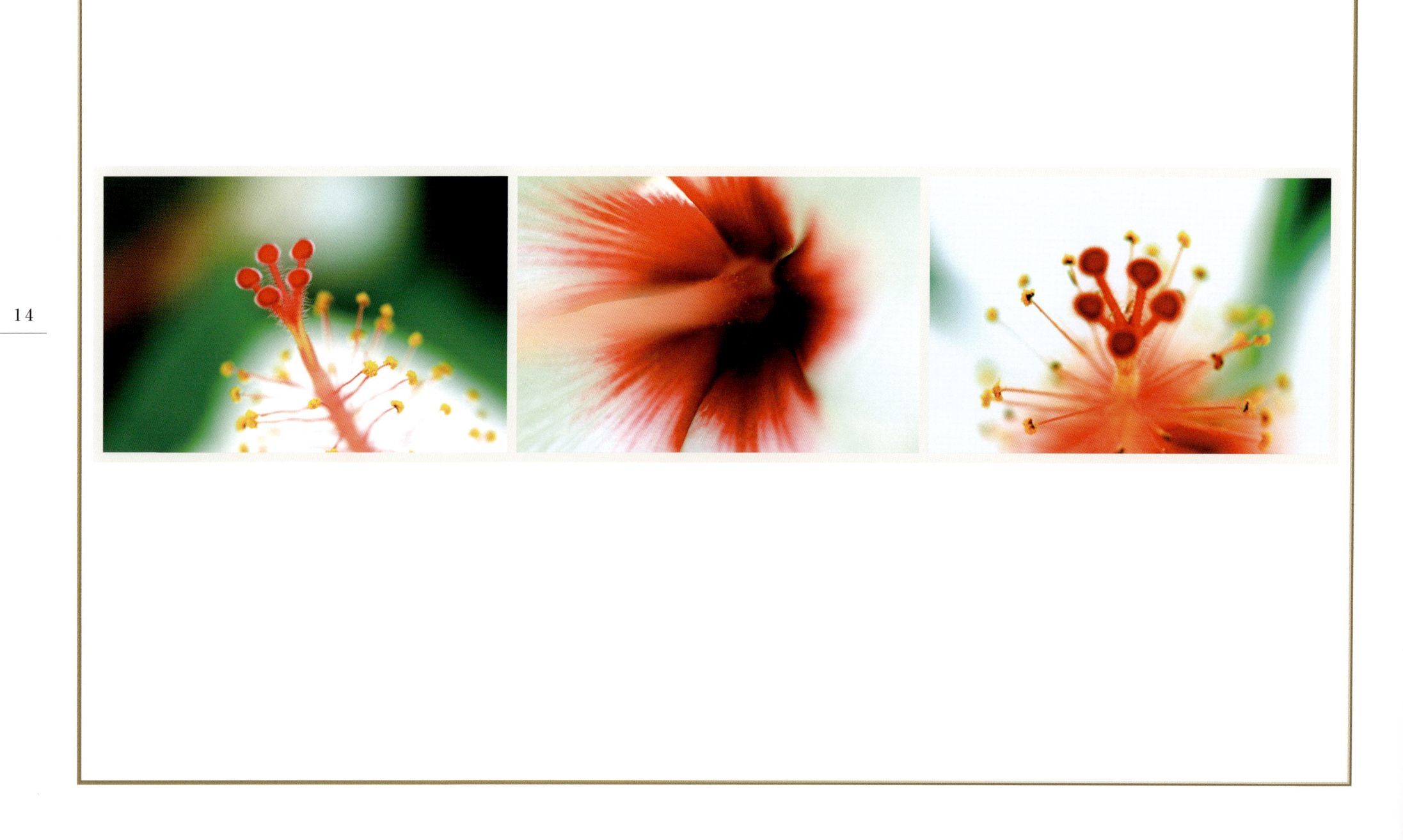

15

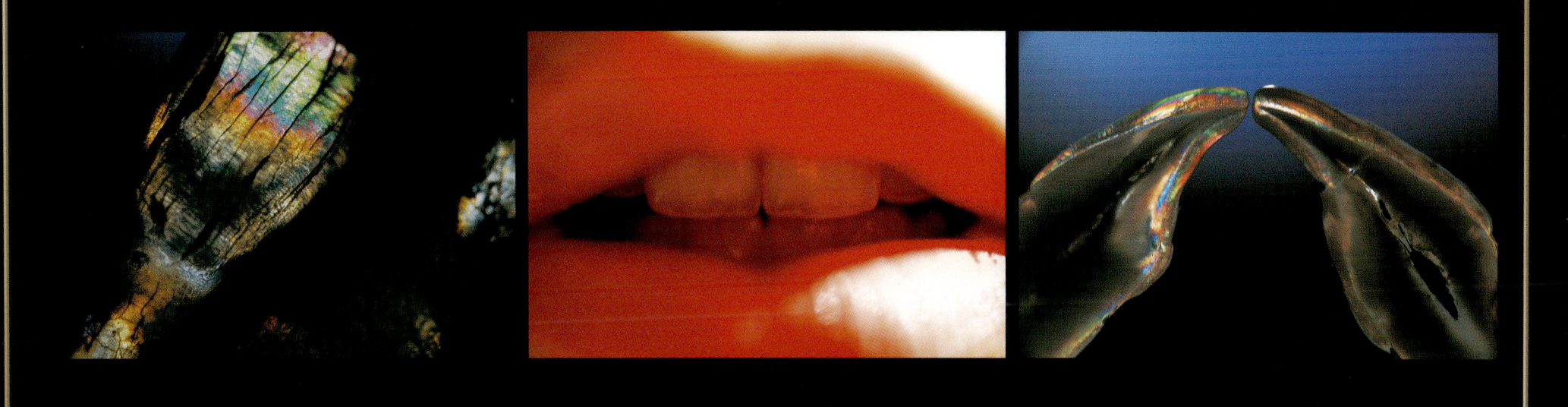

16

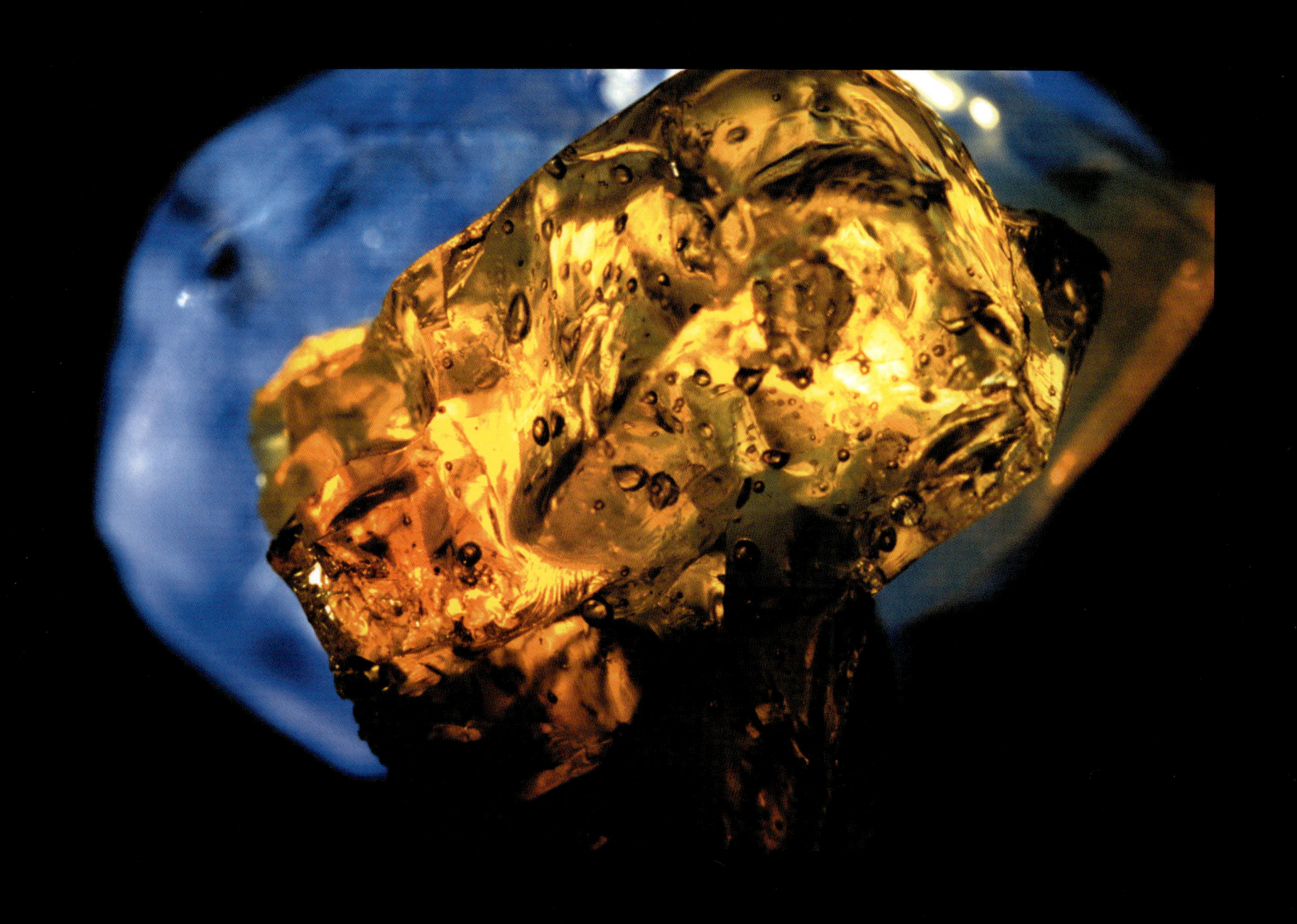

17

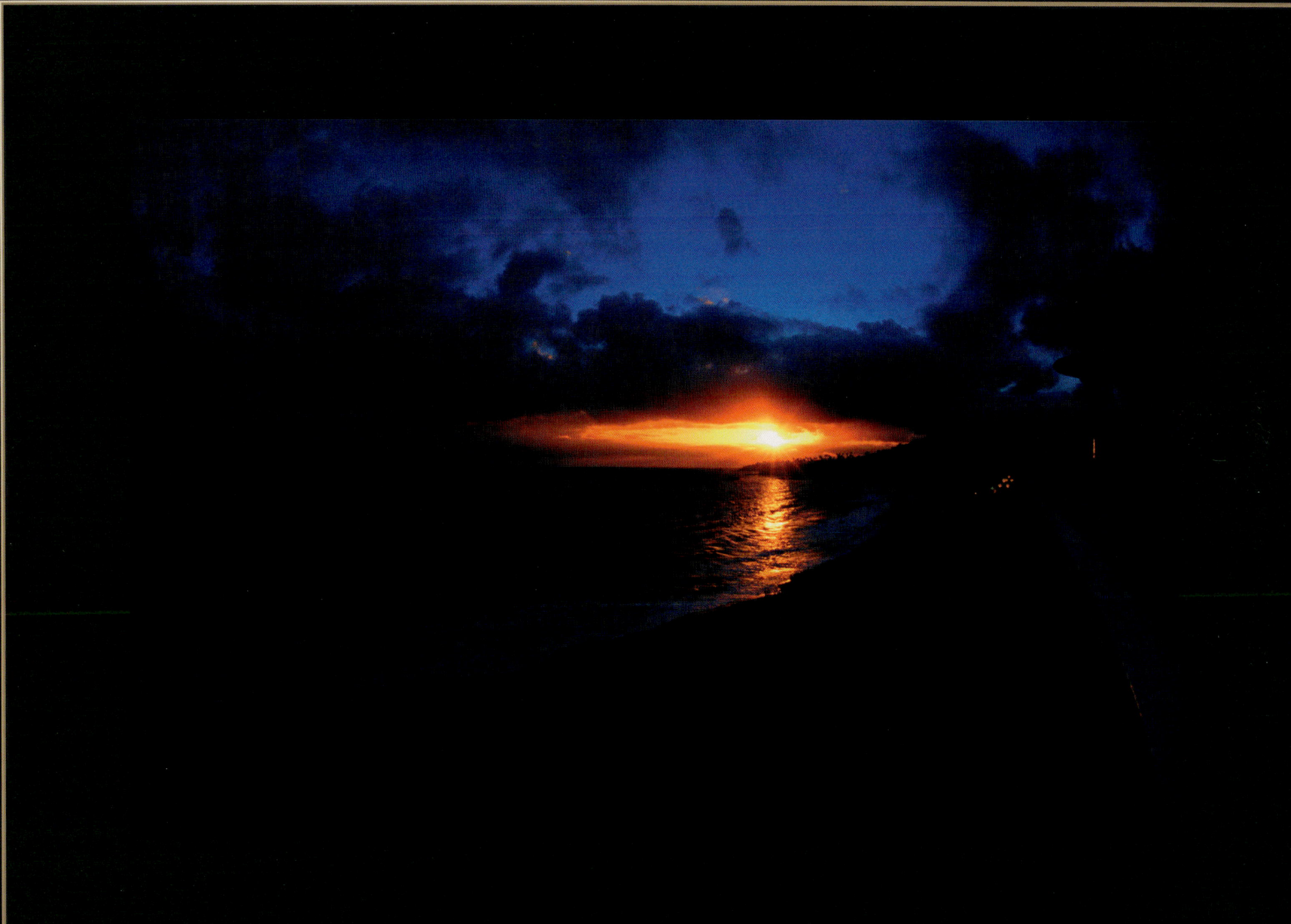

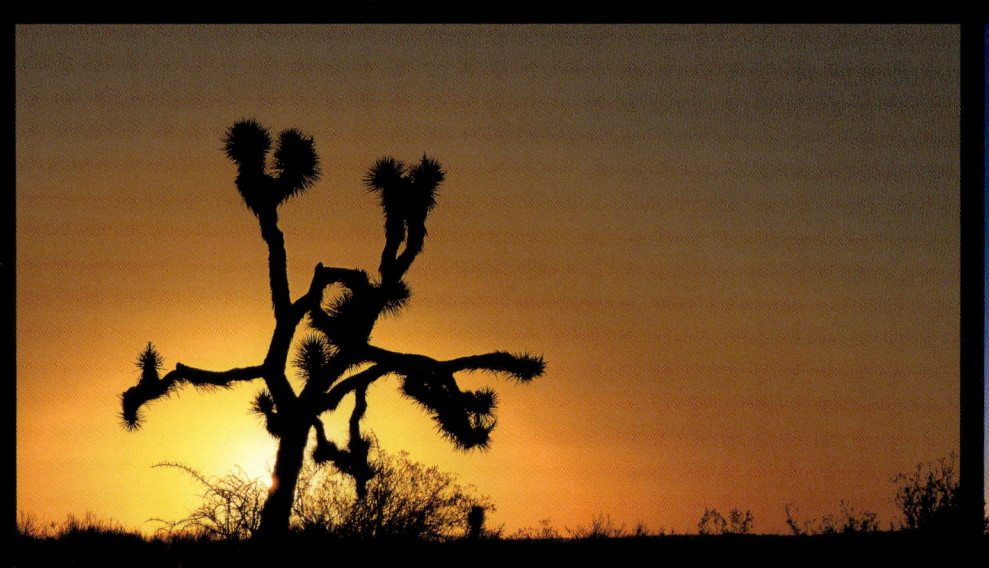

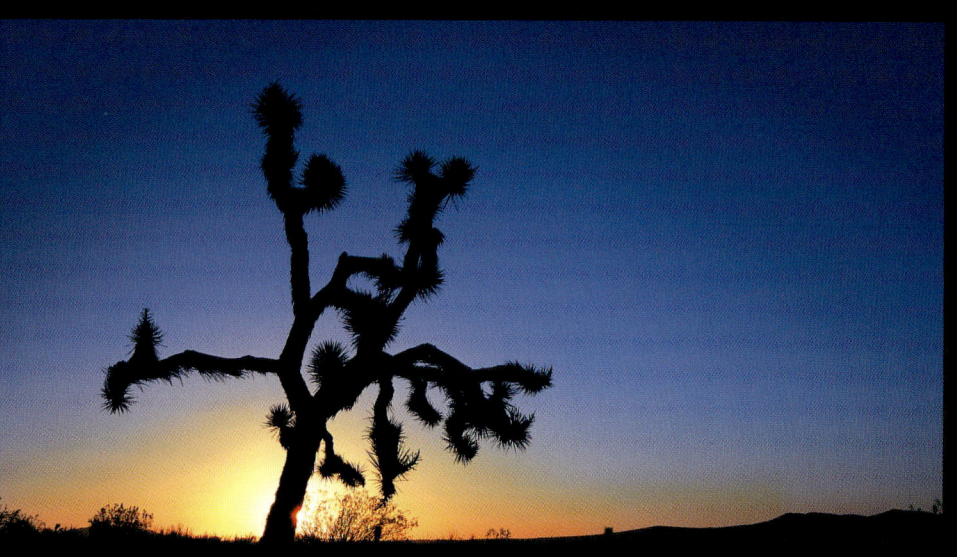

19

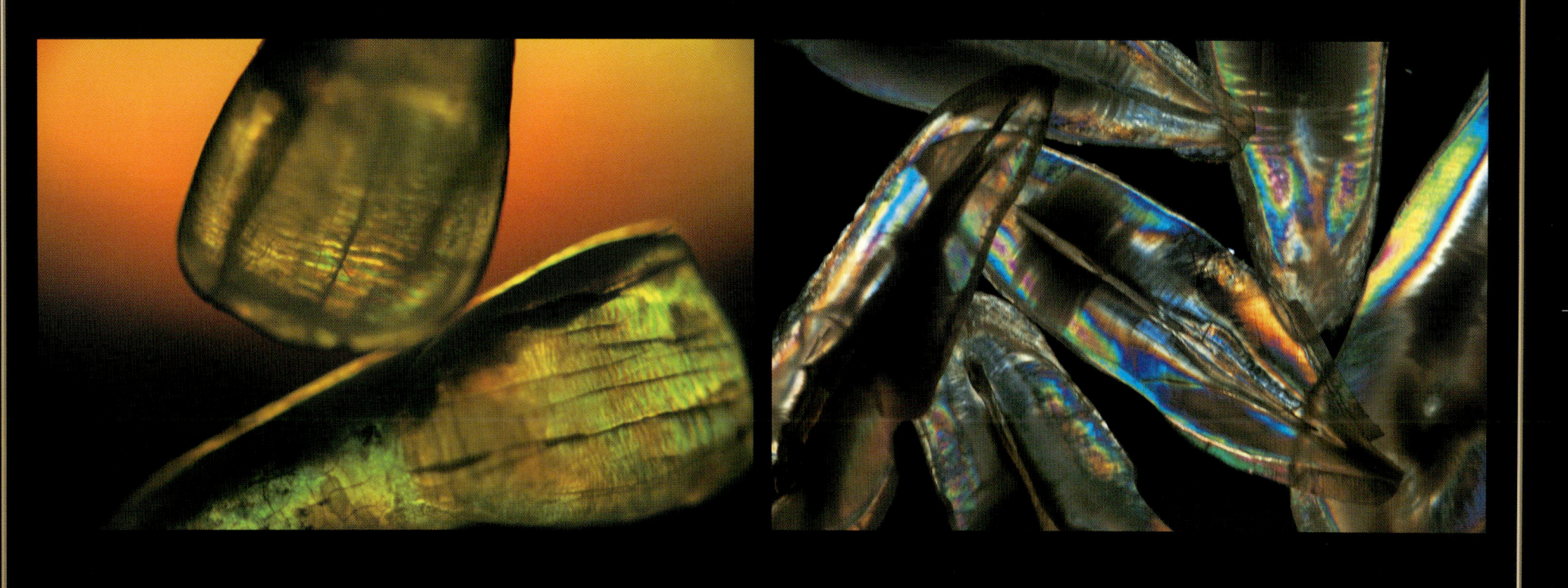

20

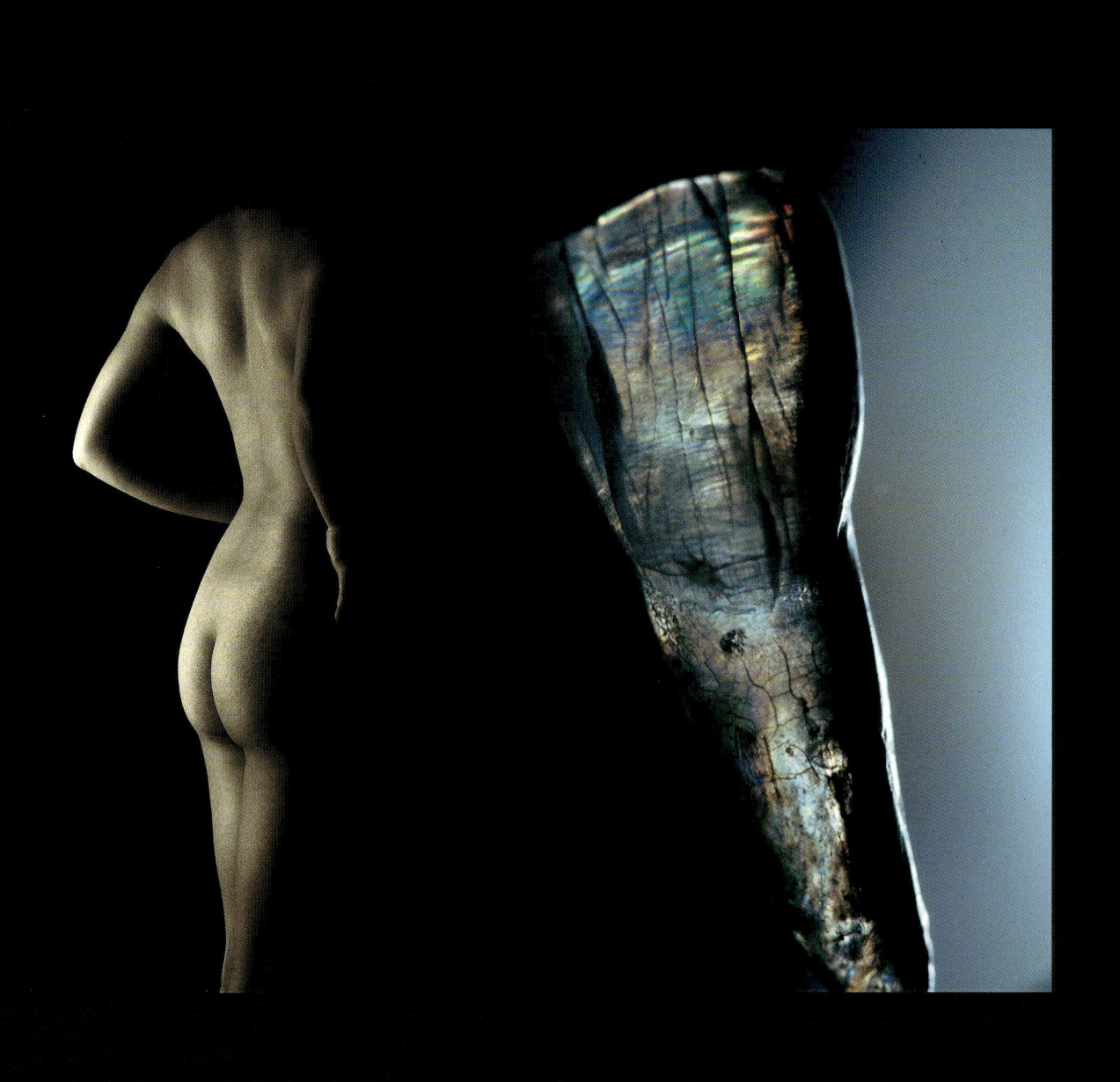

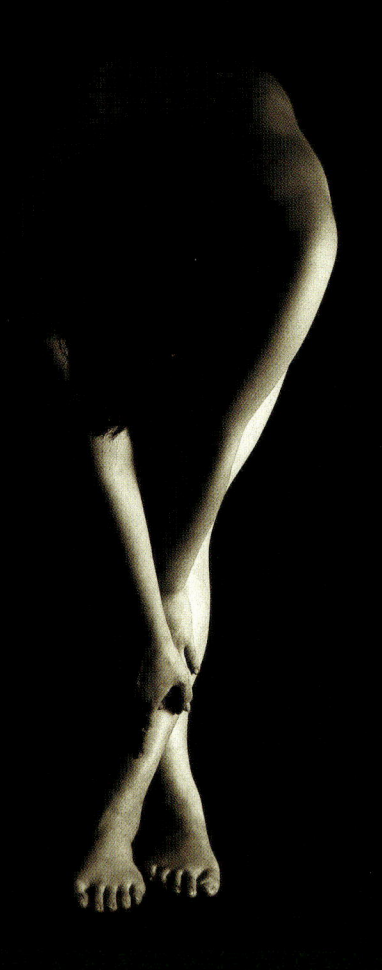

21

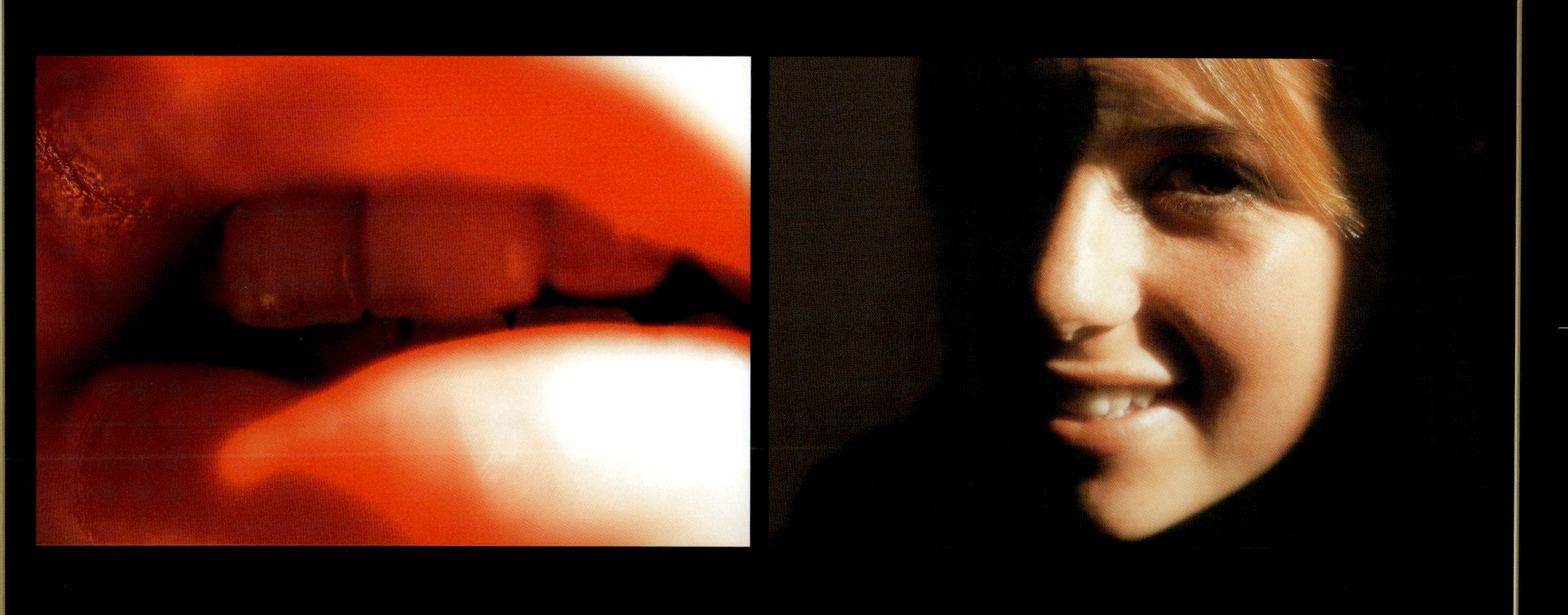

22

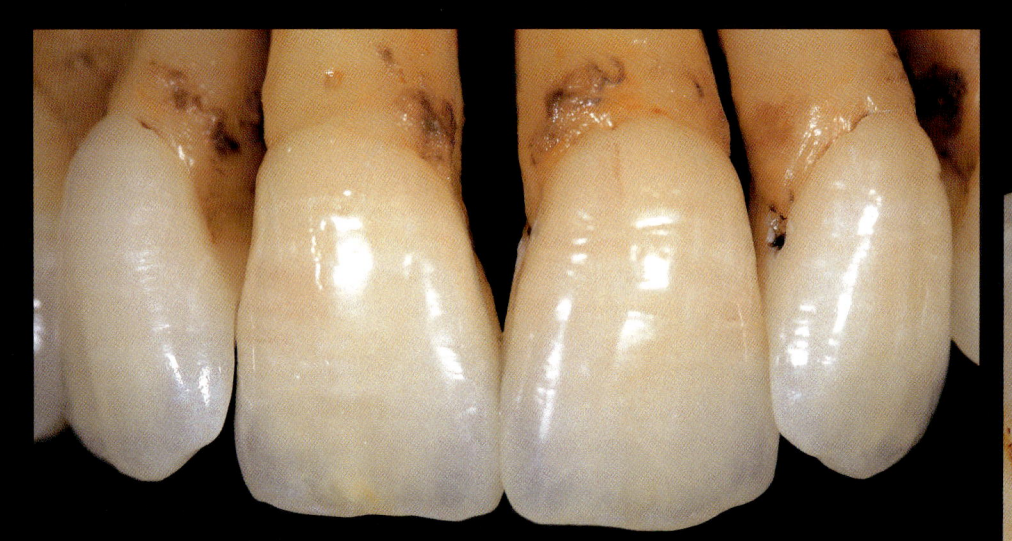

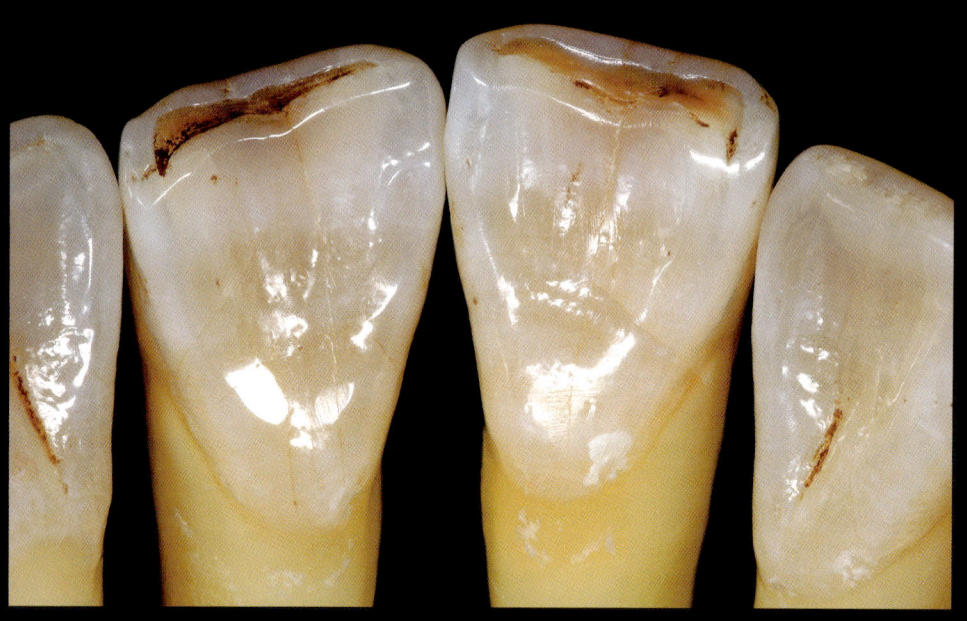

23

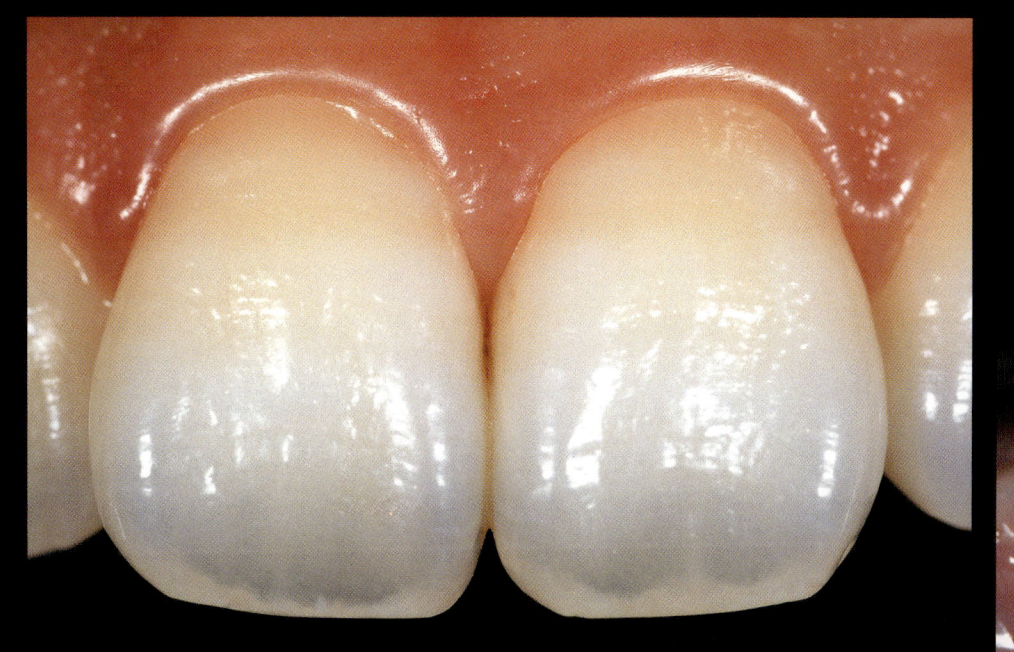

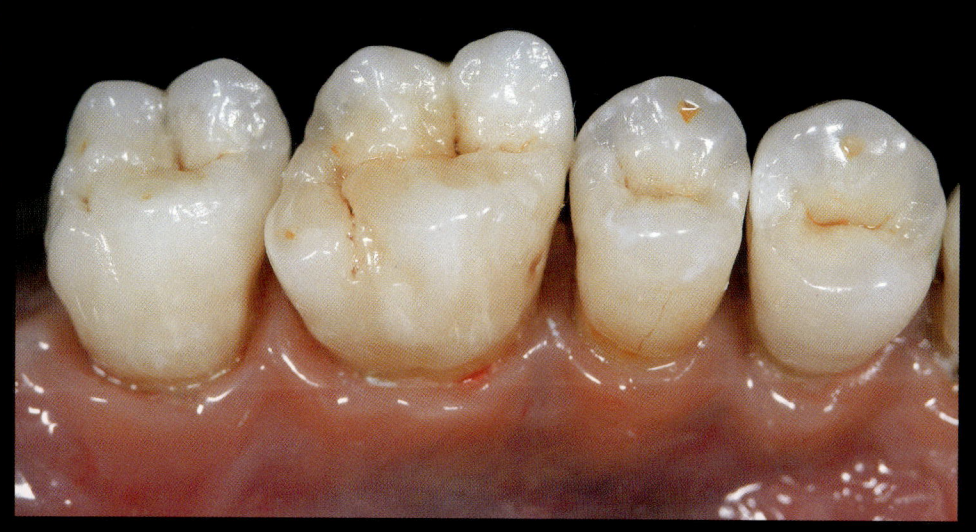

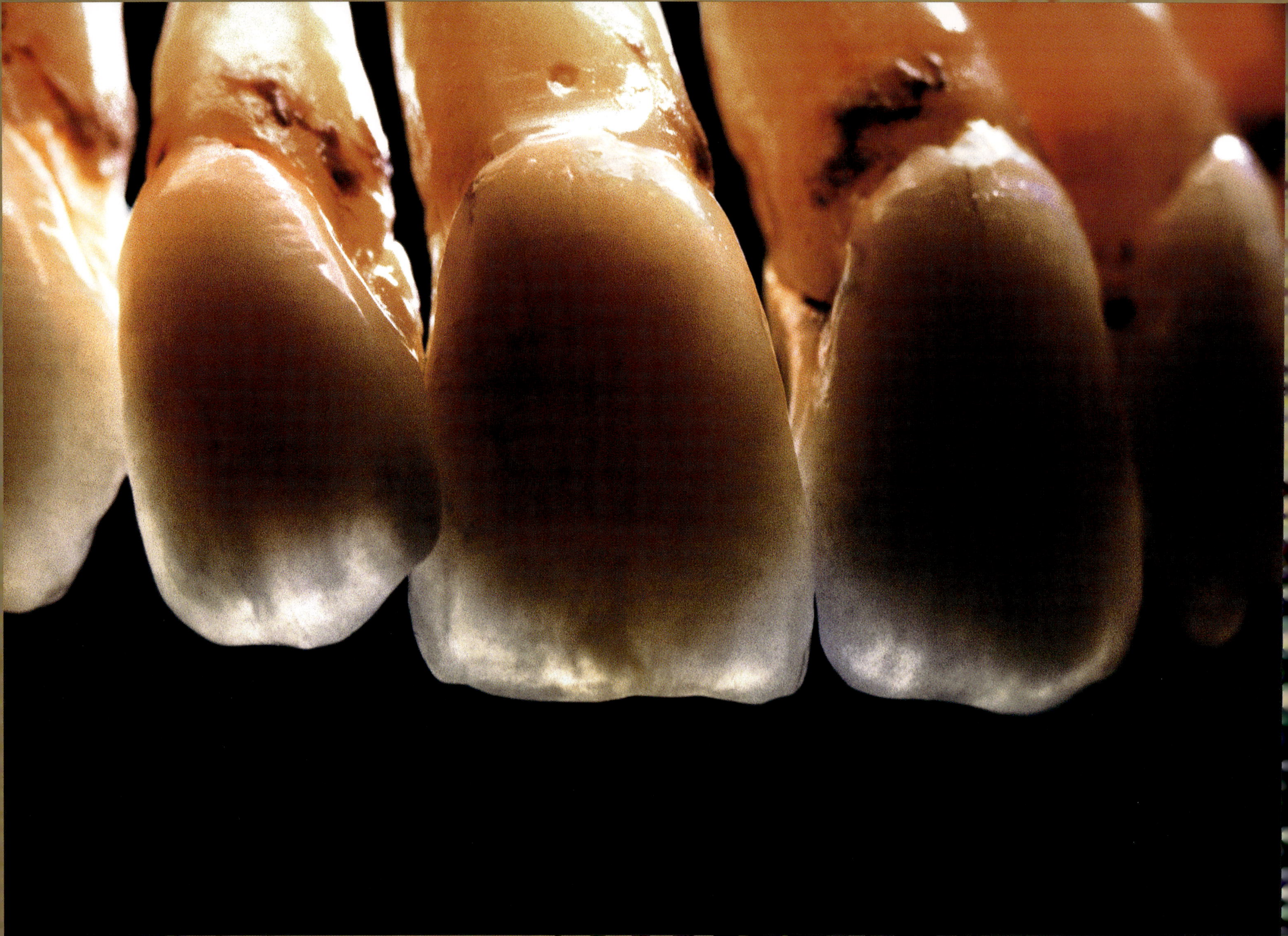

Chapter 1
Porcelain Fused Metal Crown

CASE 1

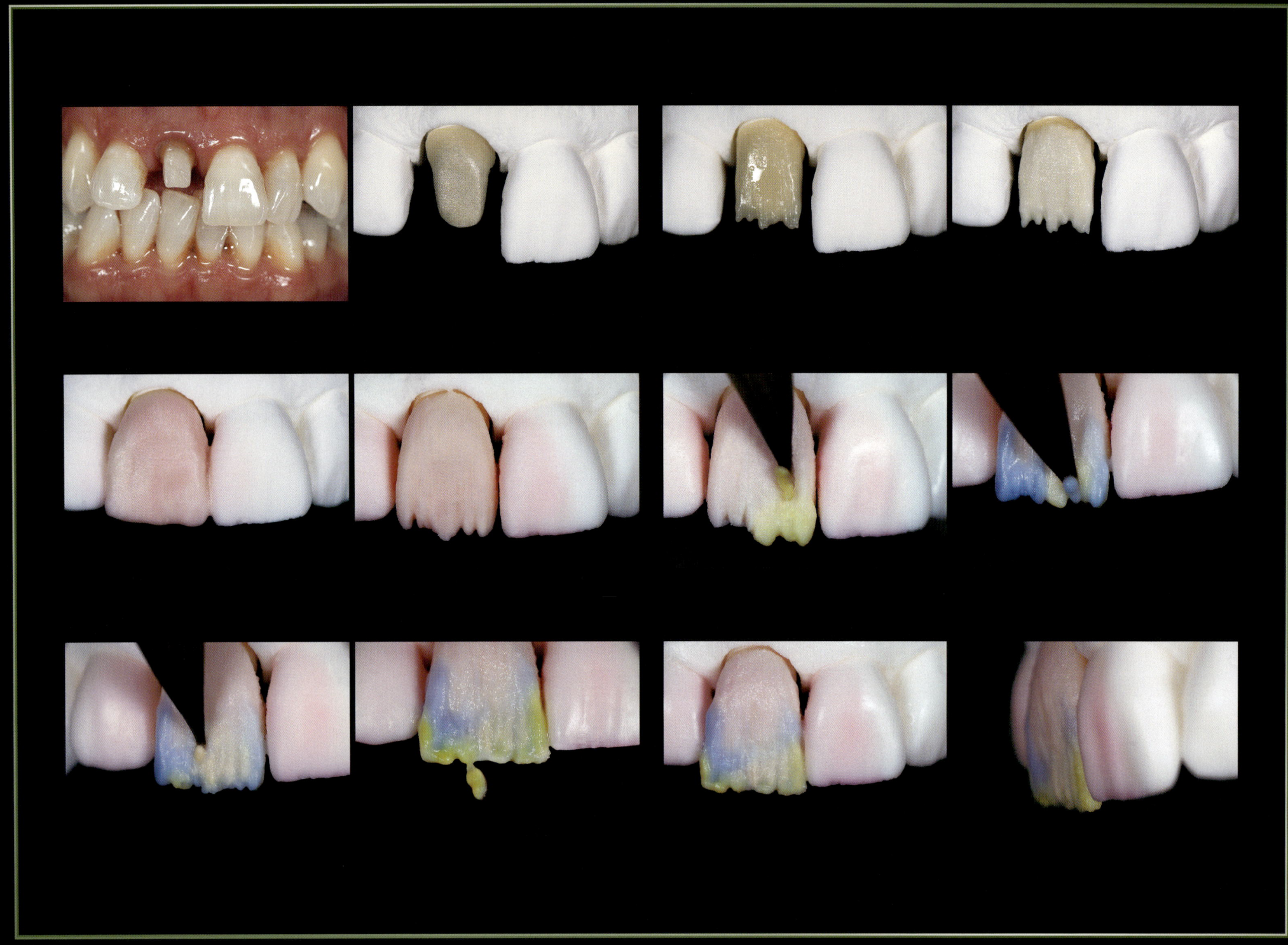

CASE 1

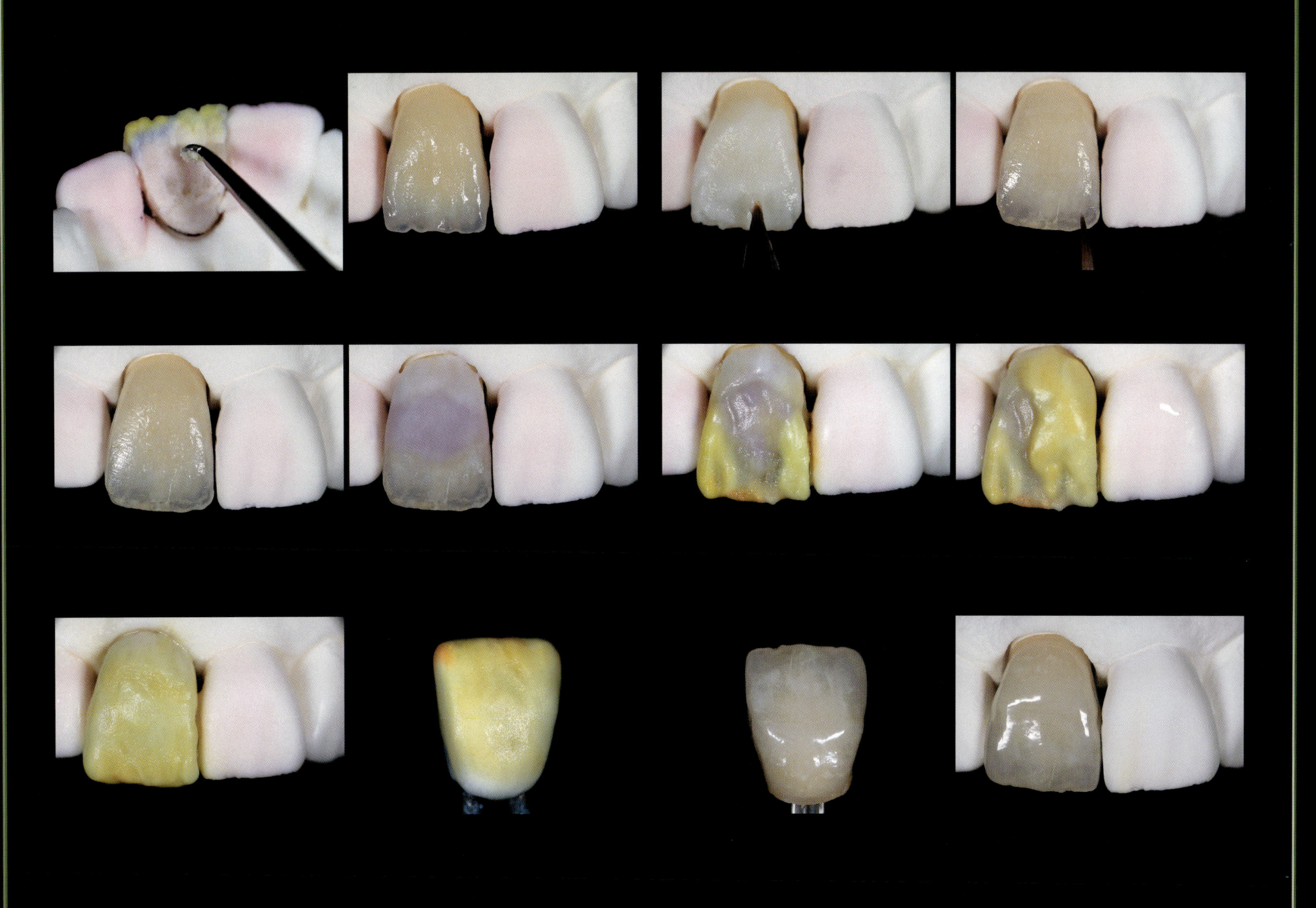

CASE 1

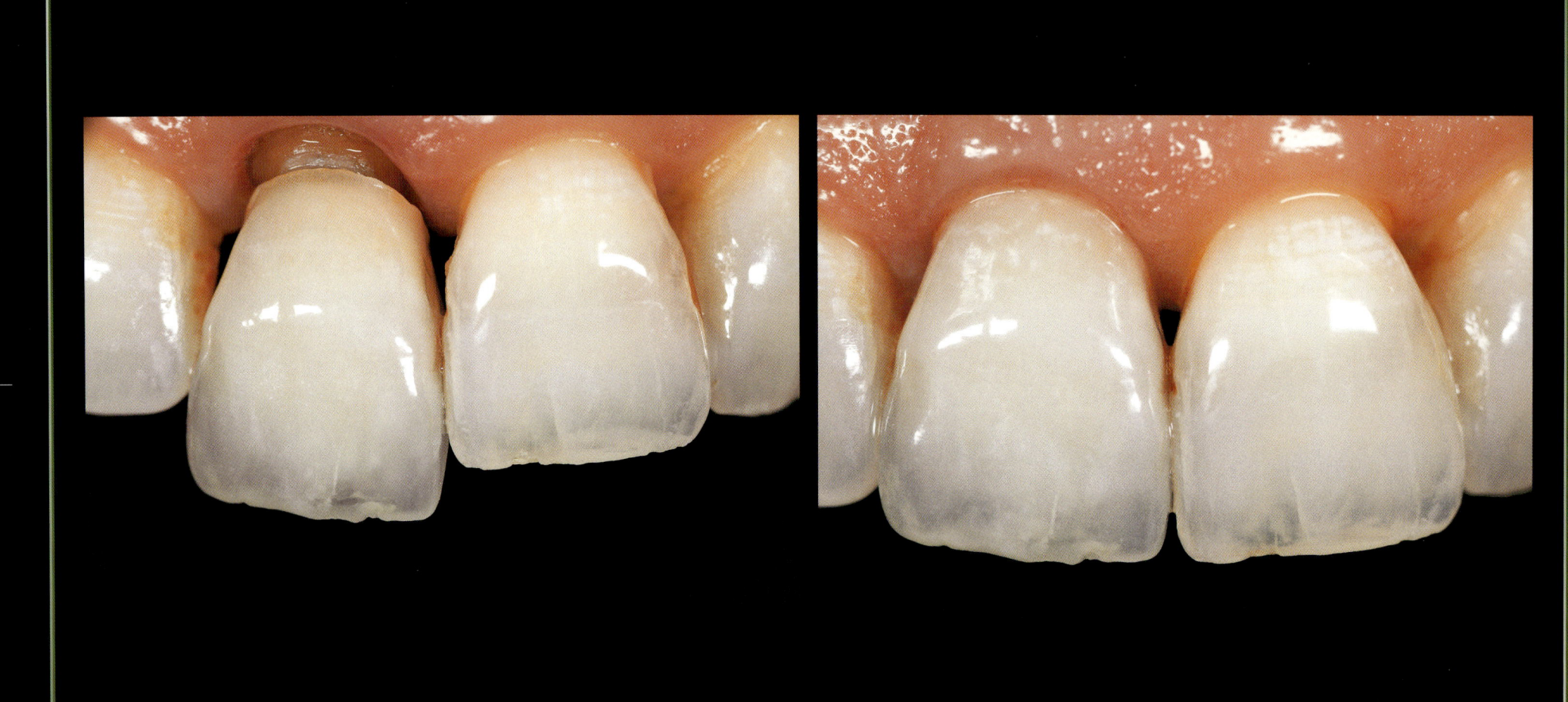

CASE 1

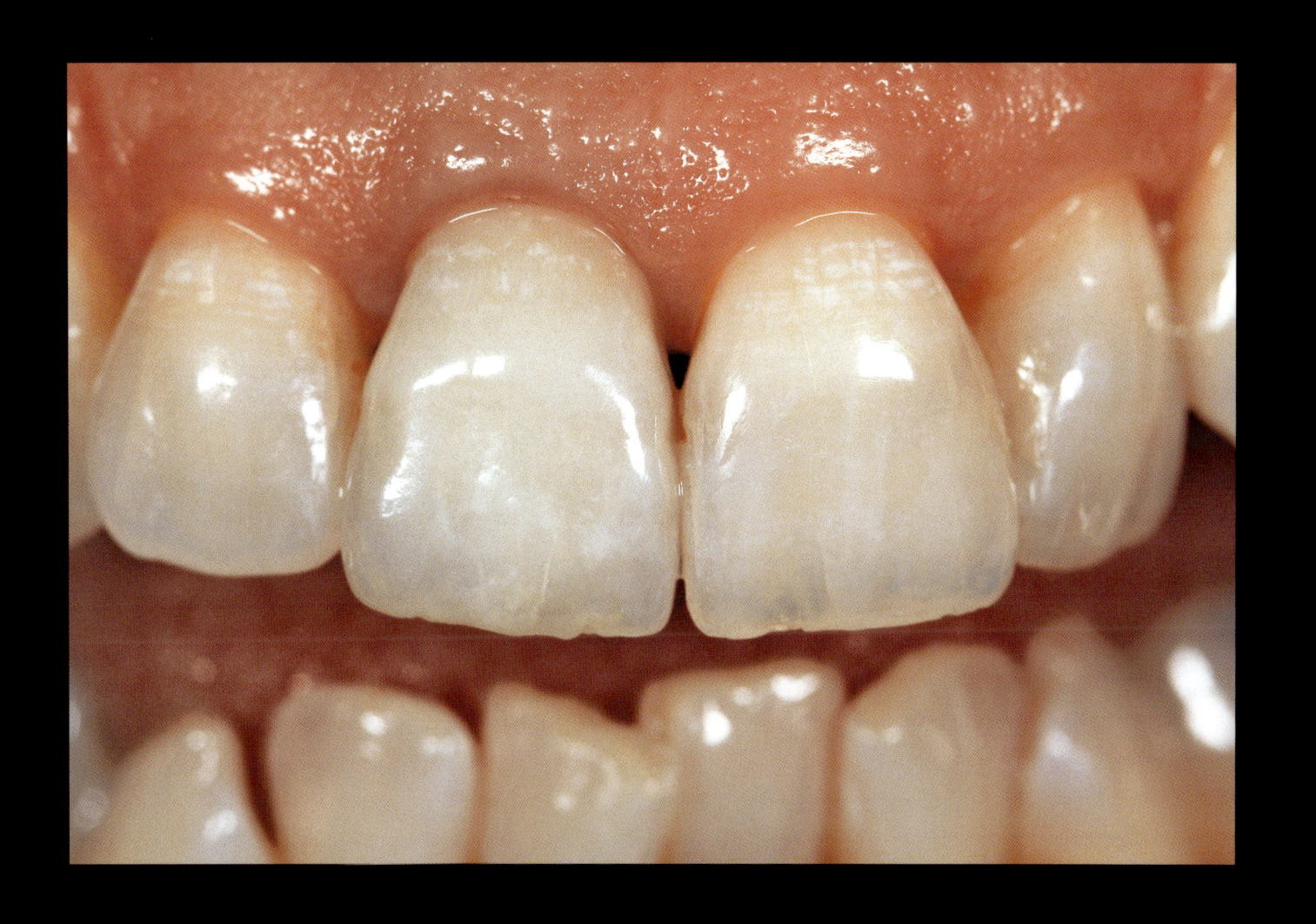

CASE 2

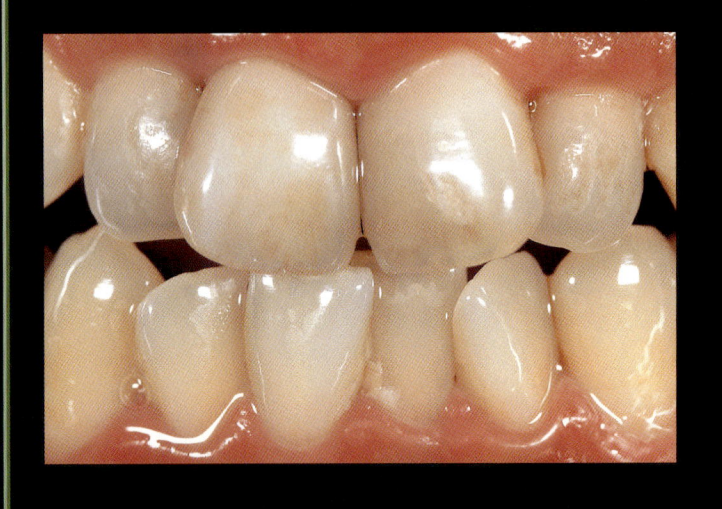

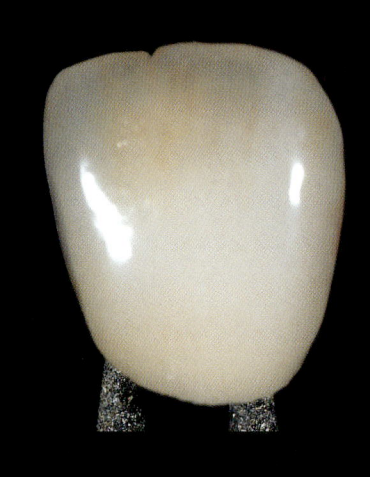

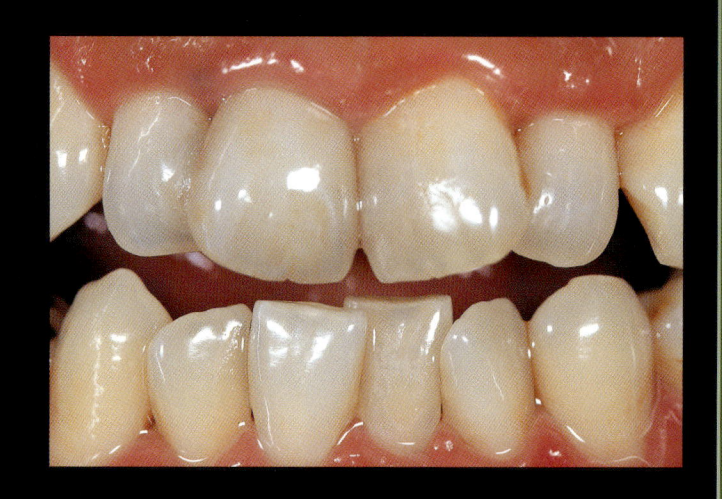

CASE 3

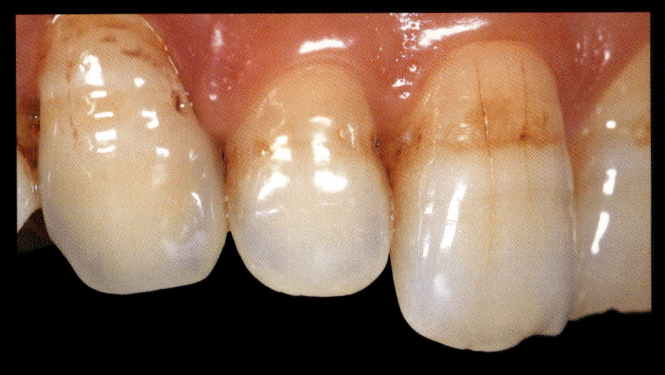

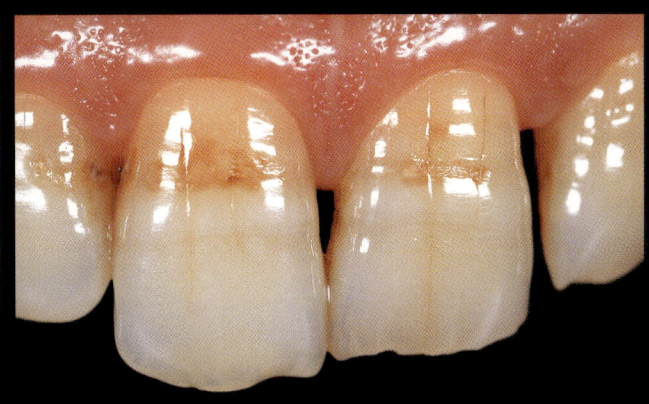

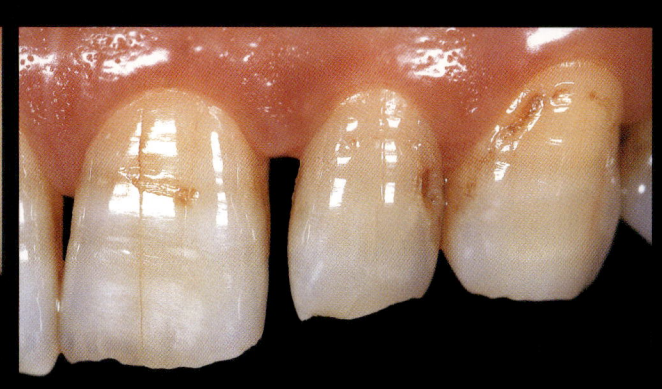

32

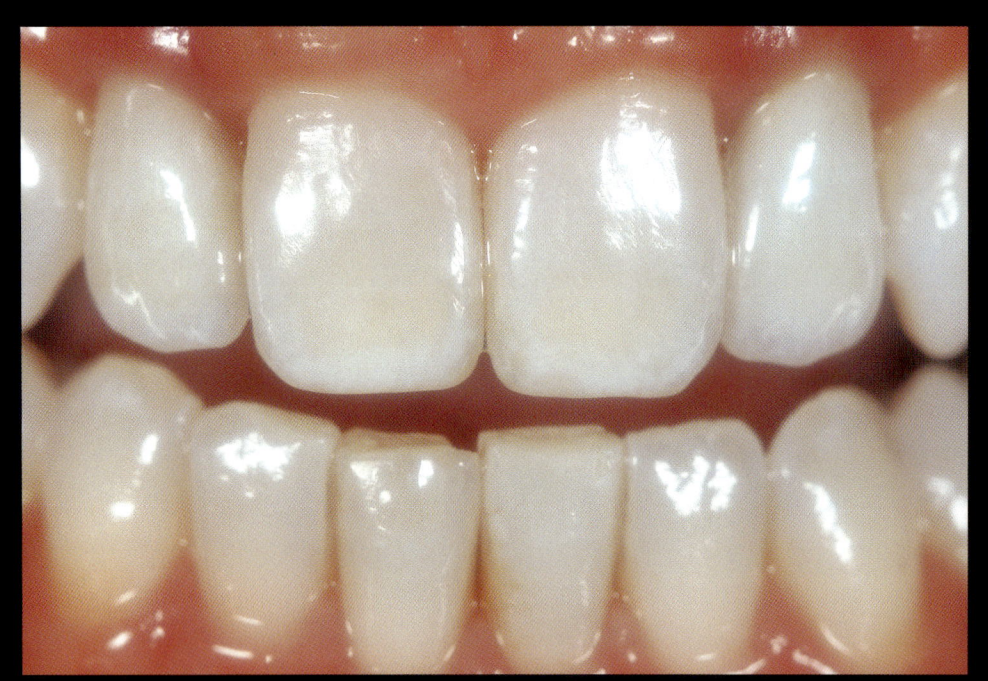

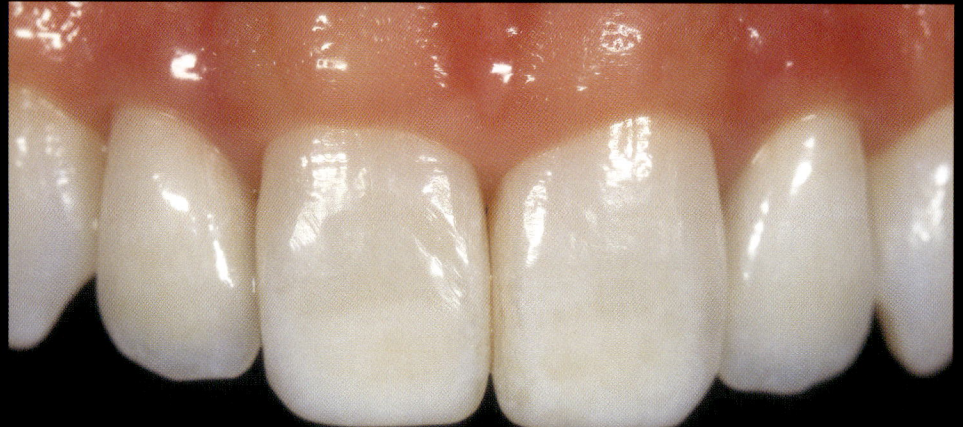

CASE 4

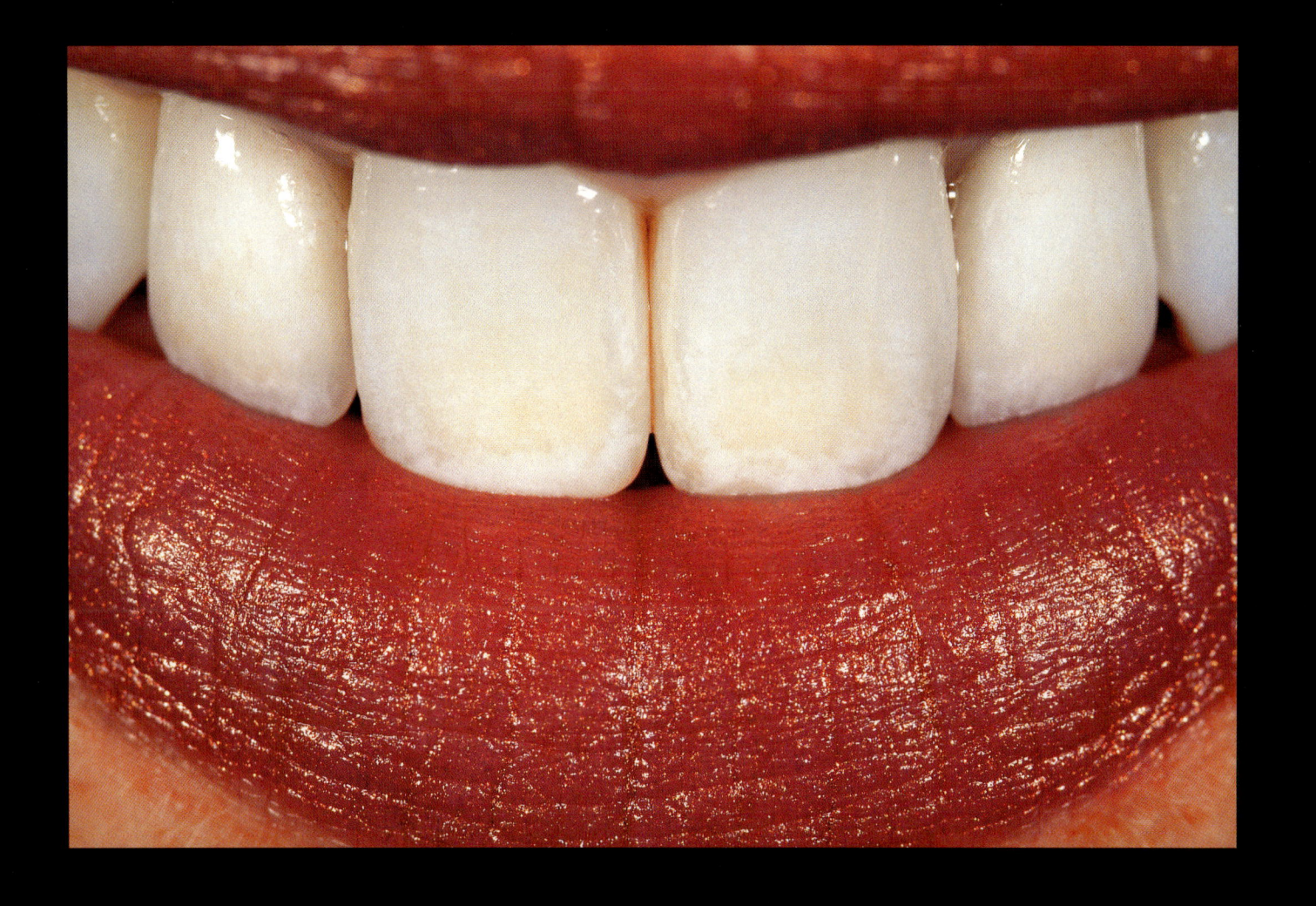

CASE 5

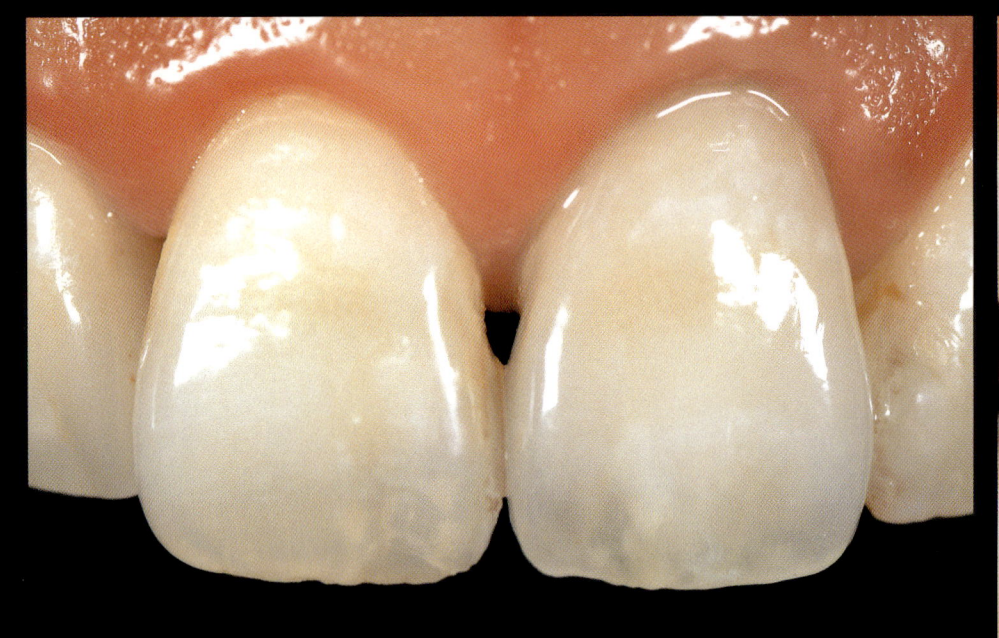

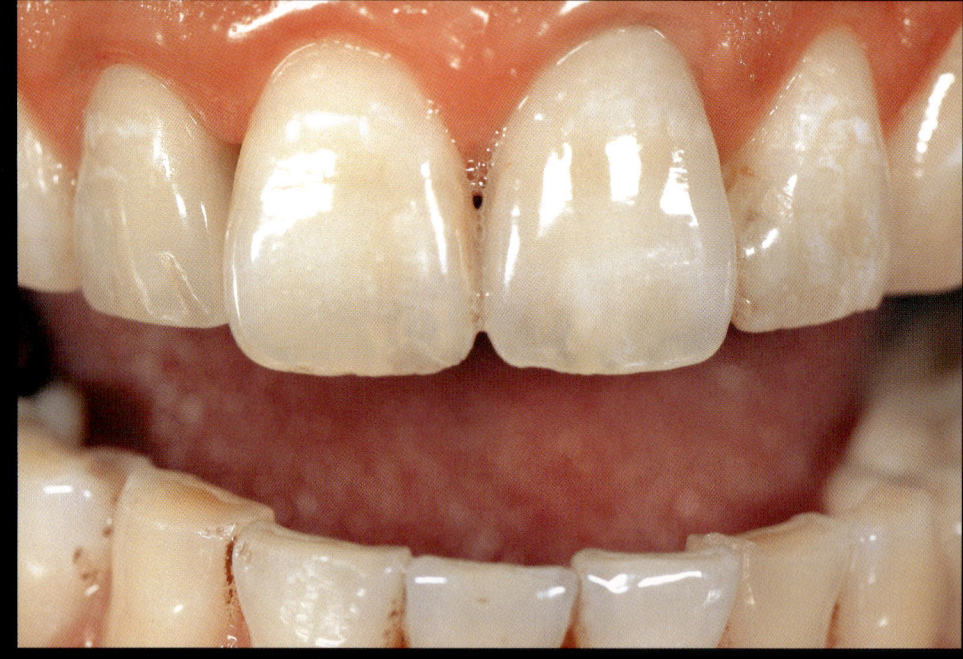

CASE 5

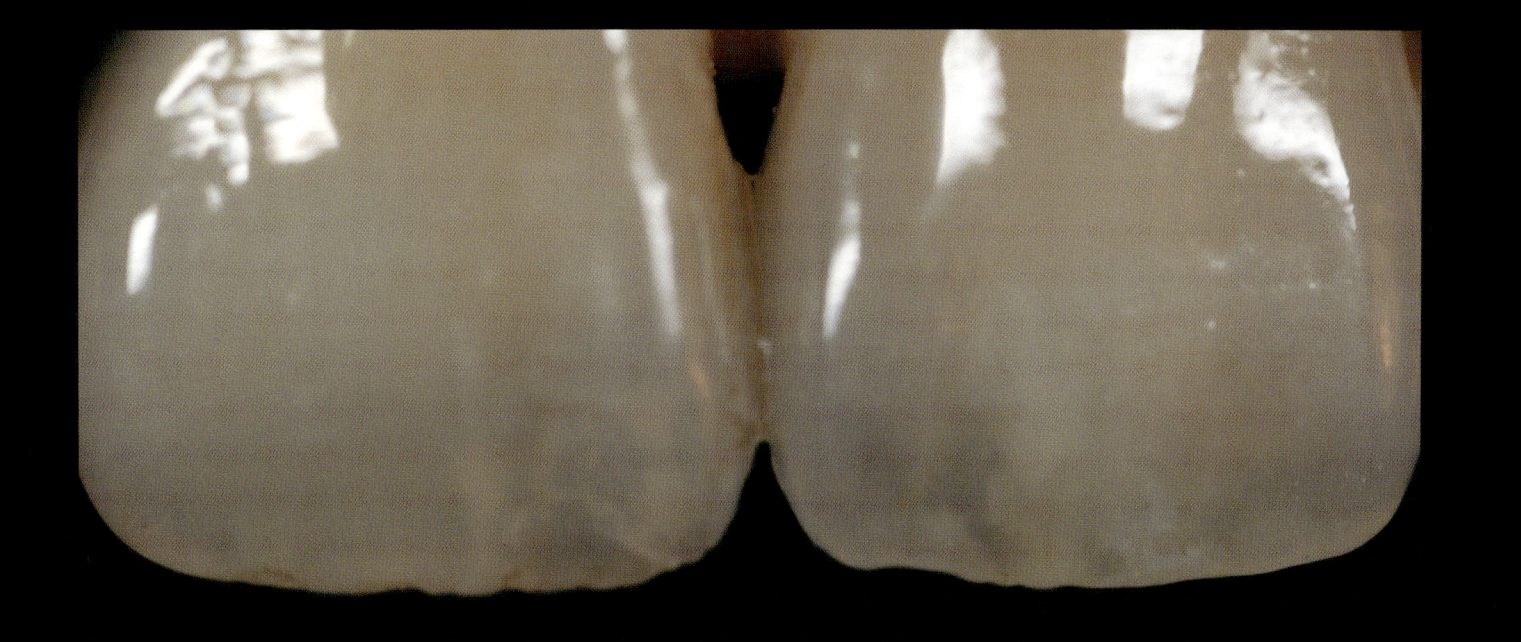

CASE 6

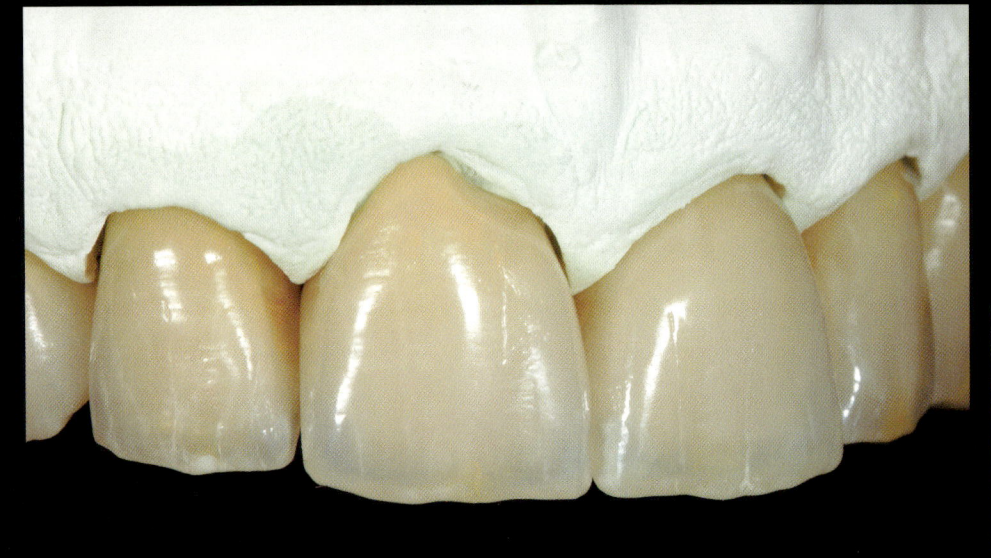

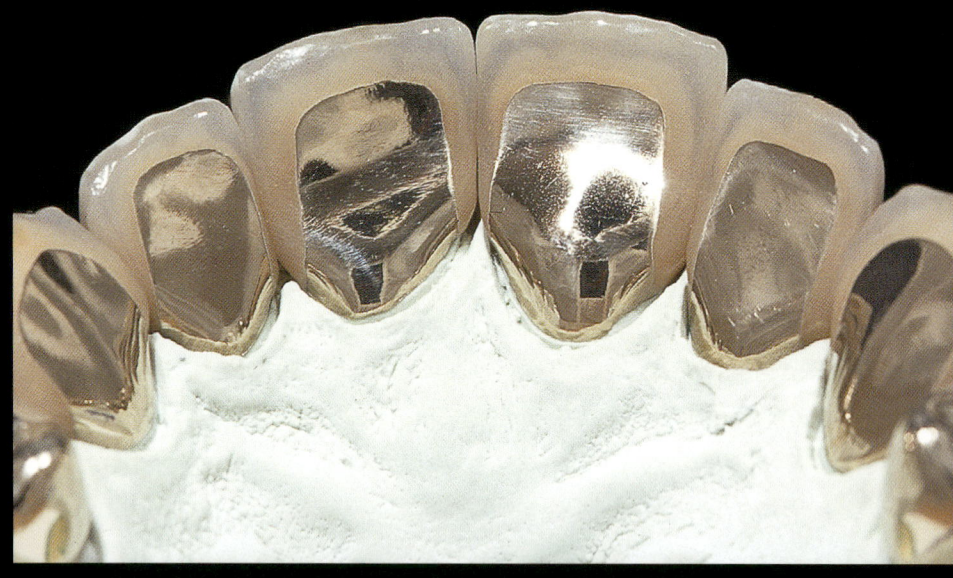

CASE 6

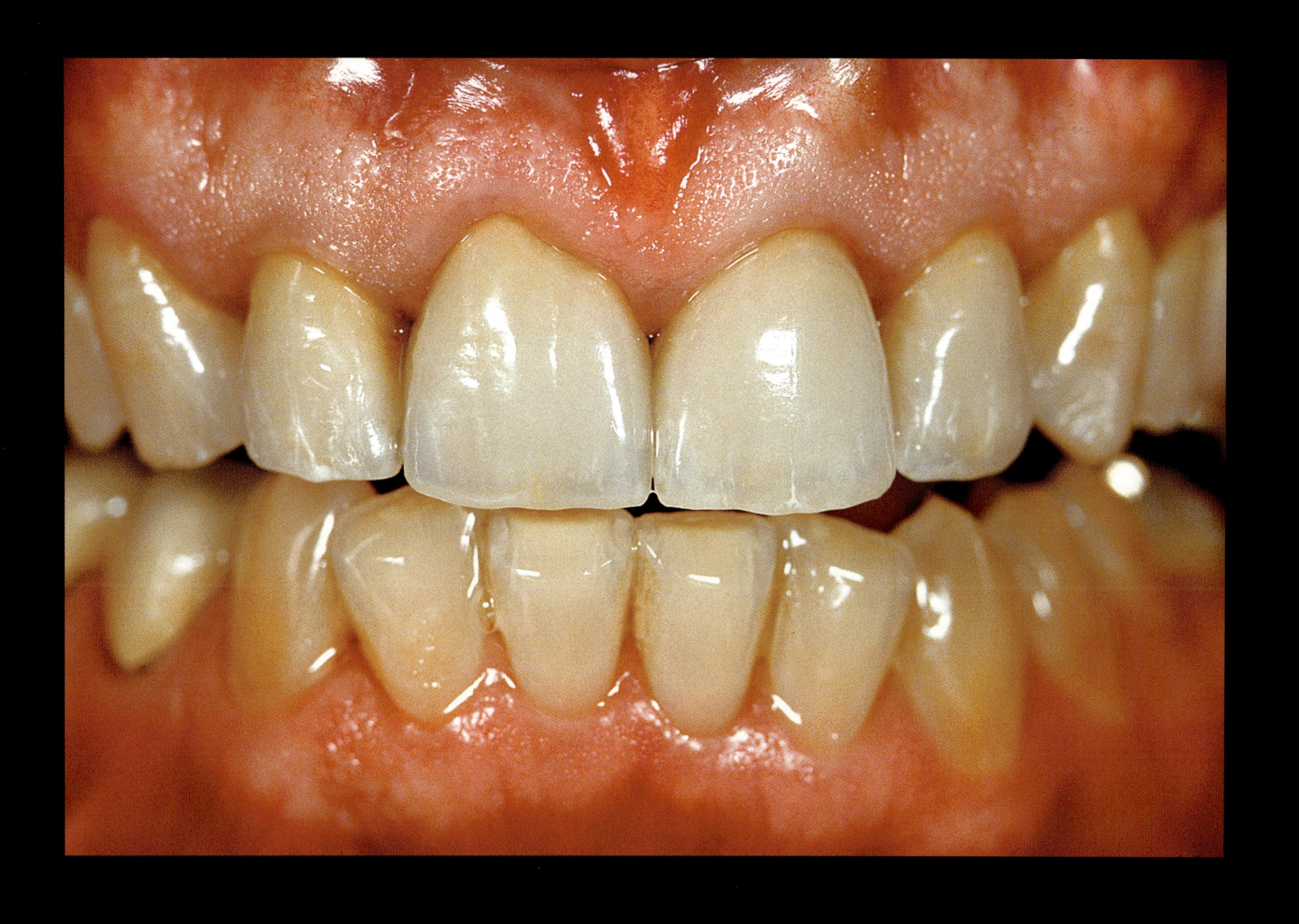

CASE 7

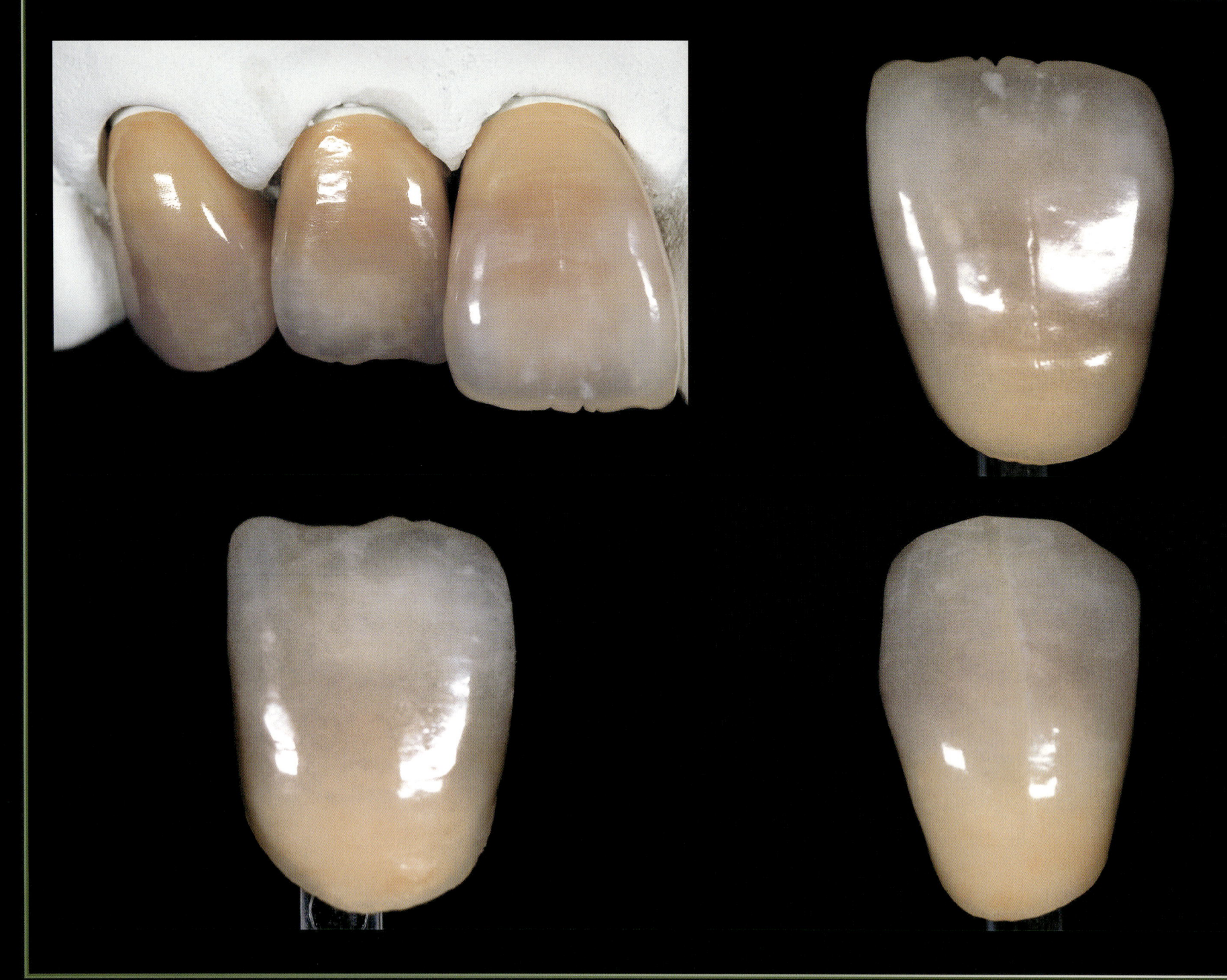

CASE 7

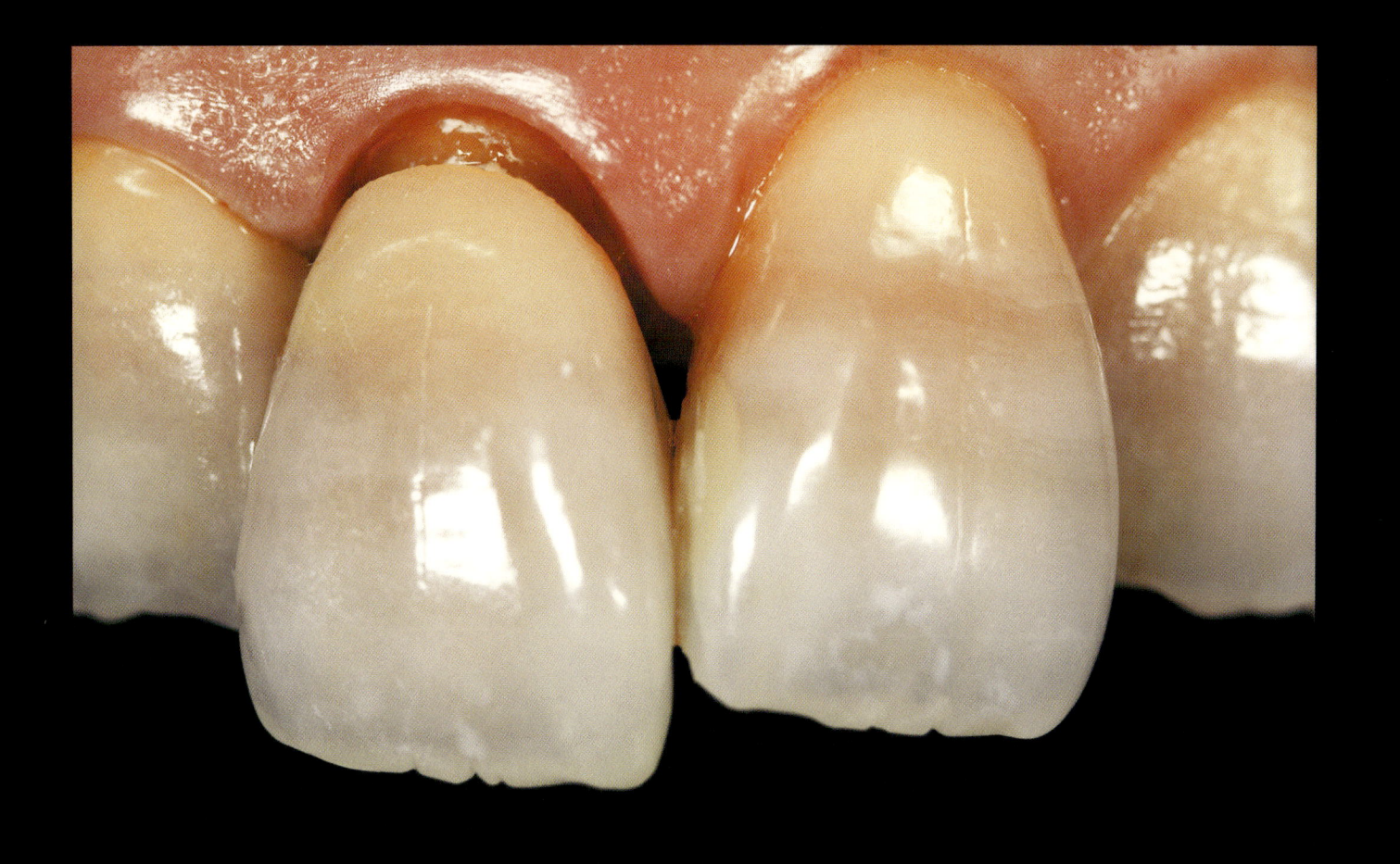

CASE 7

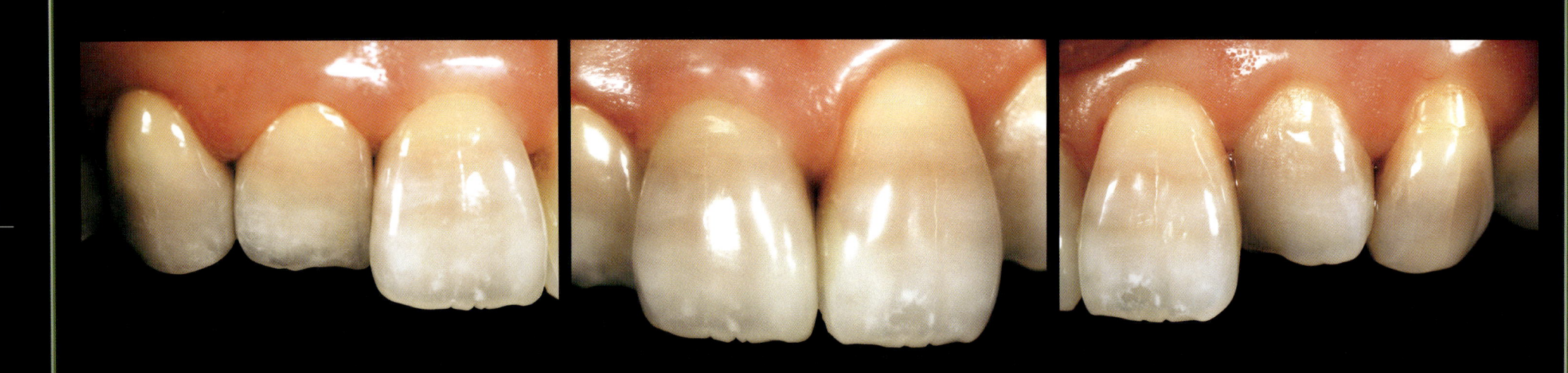

Chapter 2
All Ceramic Crown

CASE 8

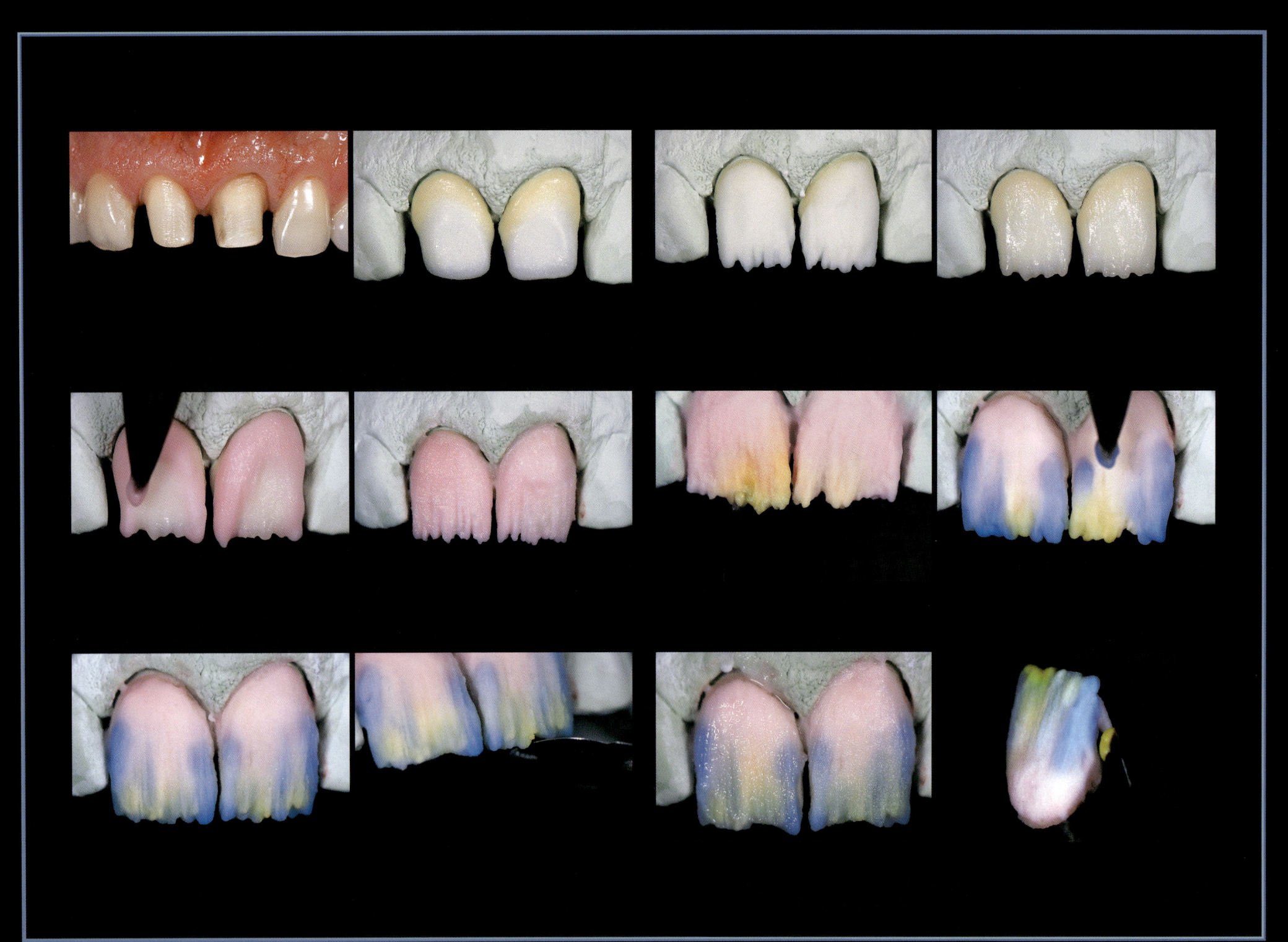

CASE 8

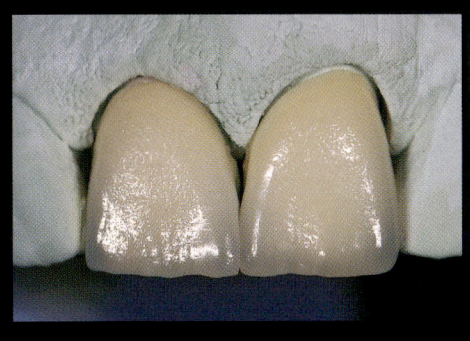

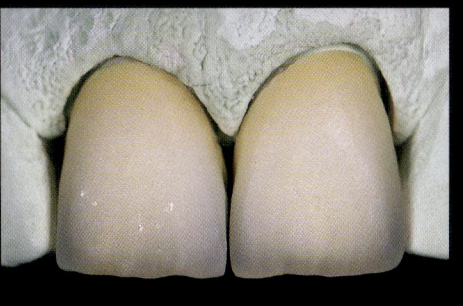

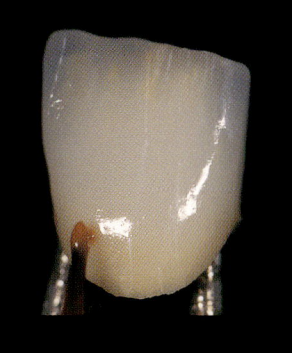

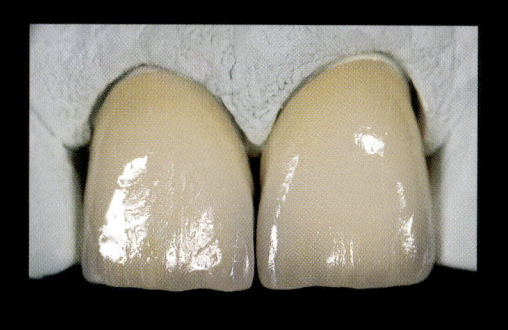

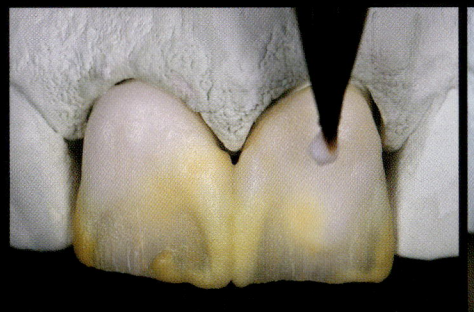

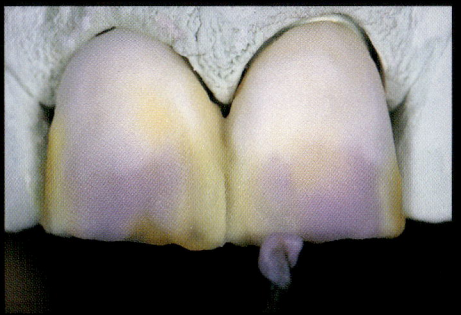

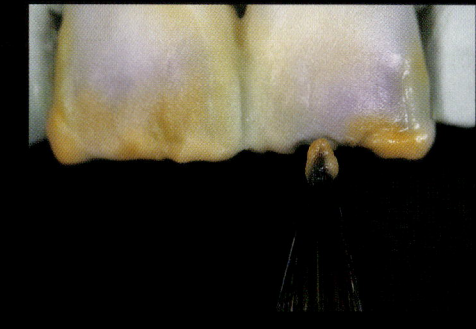

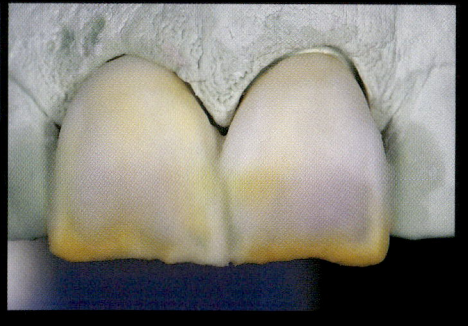

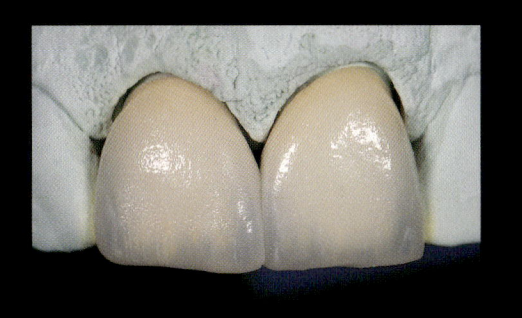

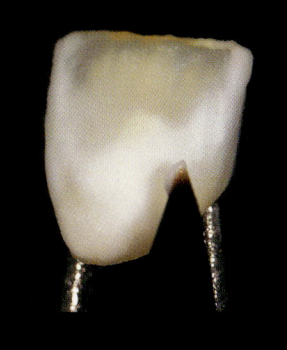

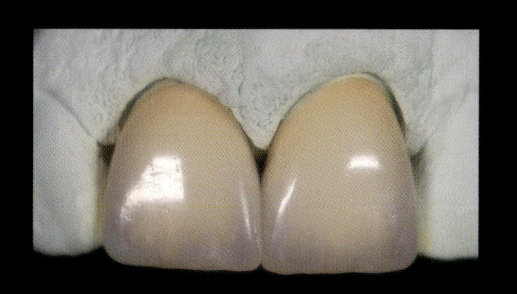

CASE 8

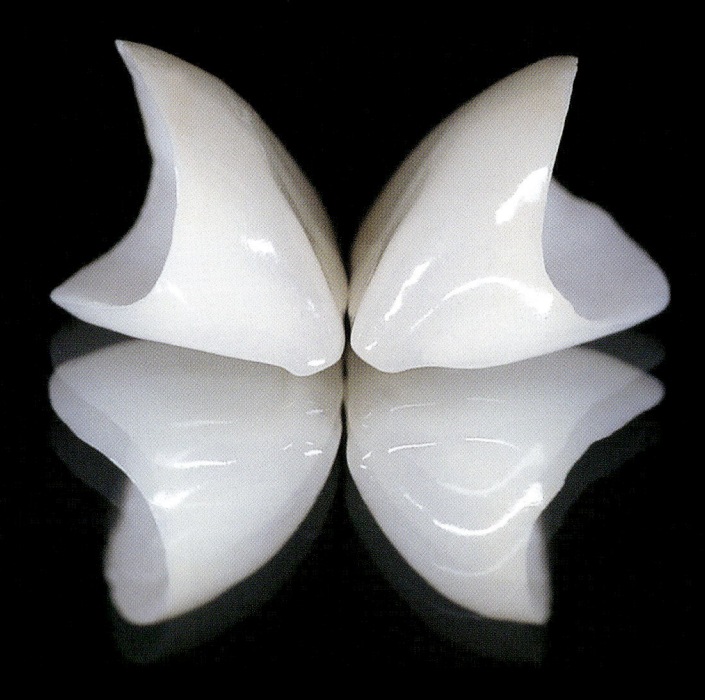

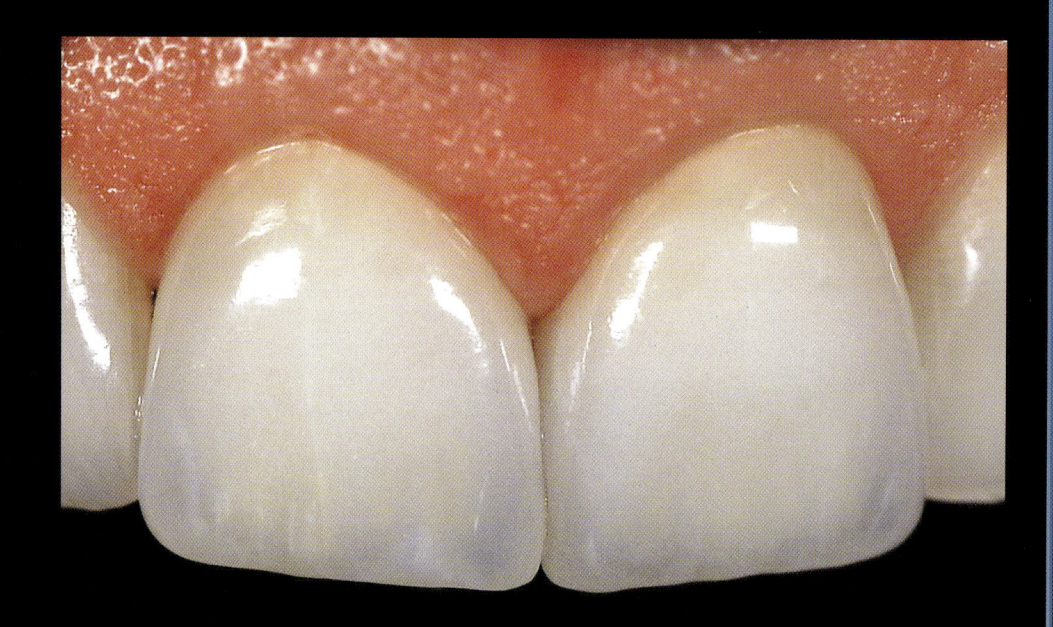

CASE 8

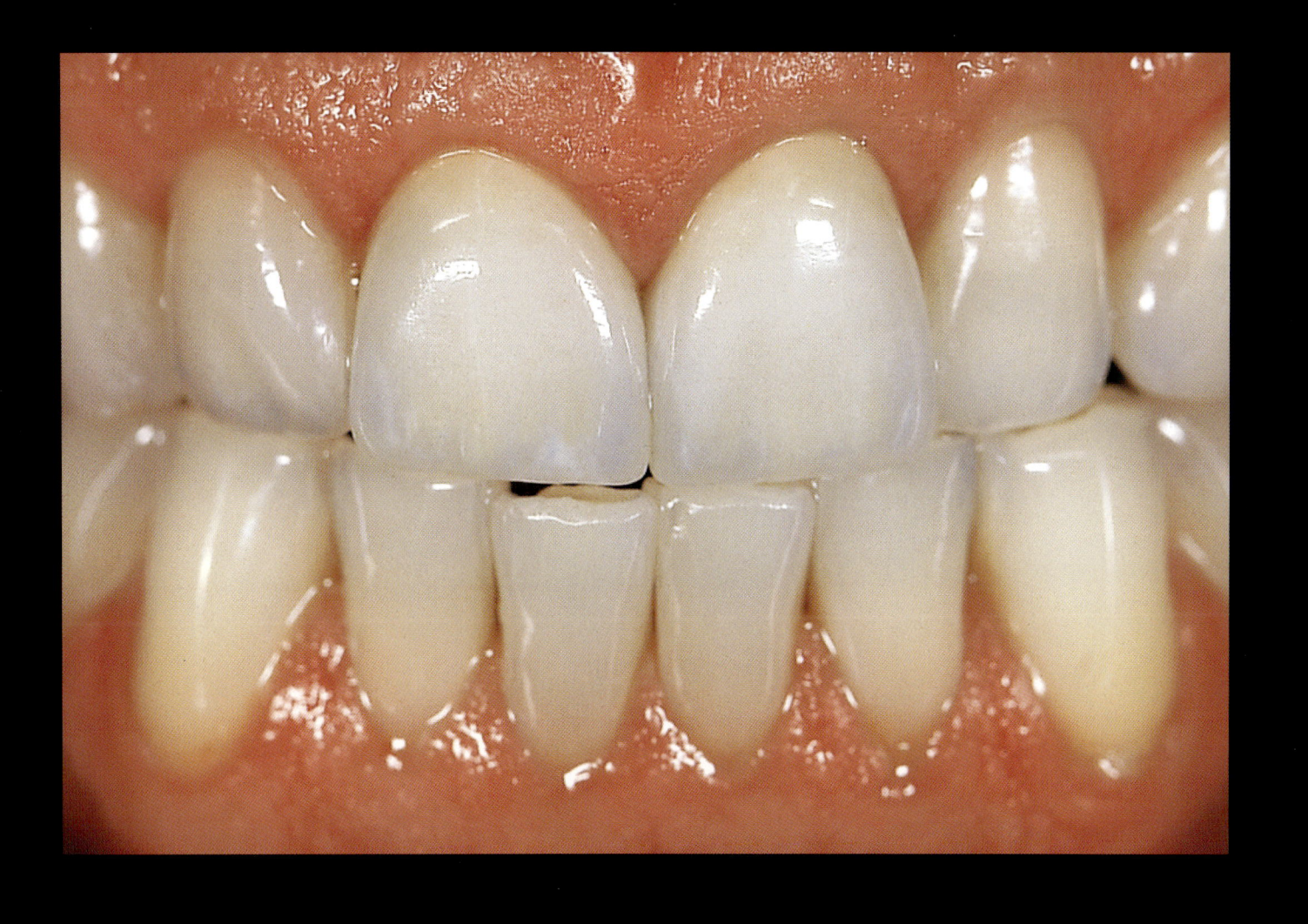

CASE 9

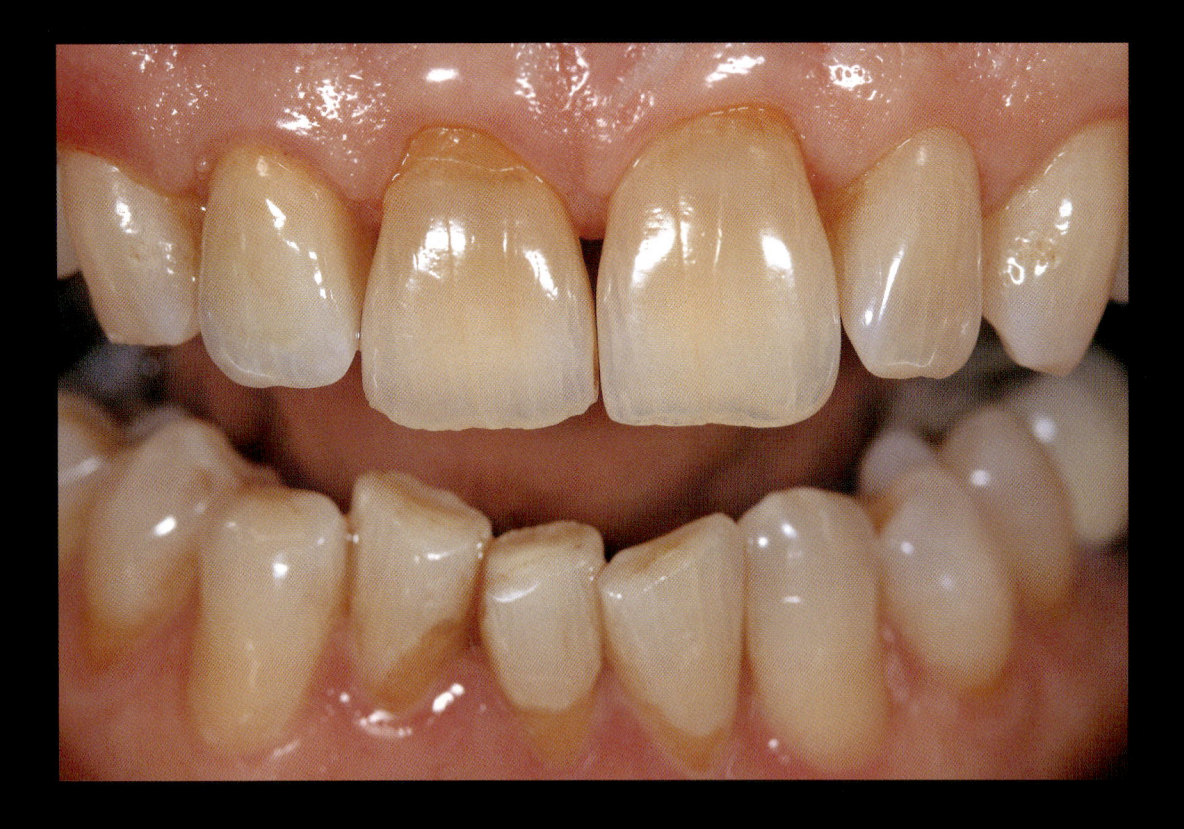

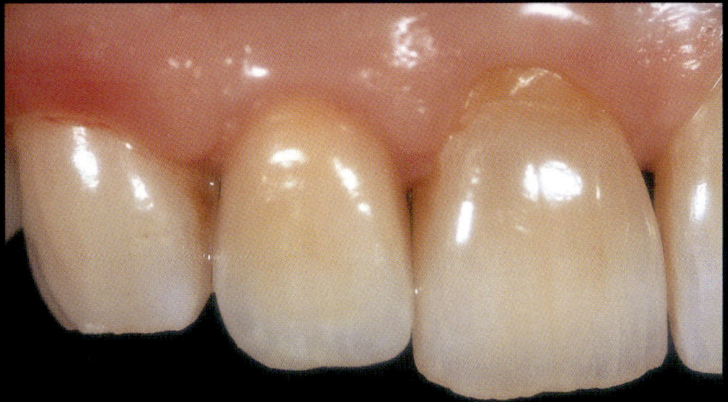
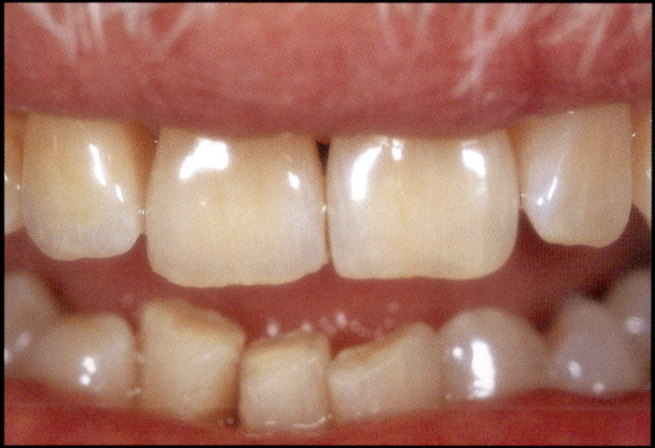
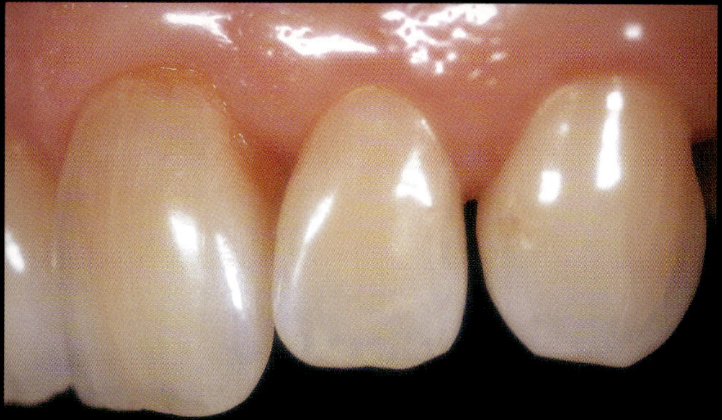

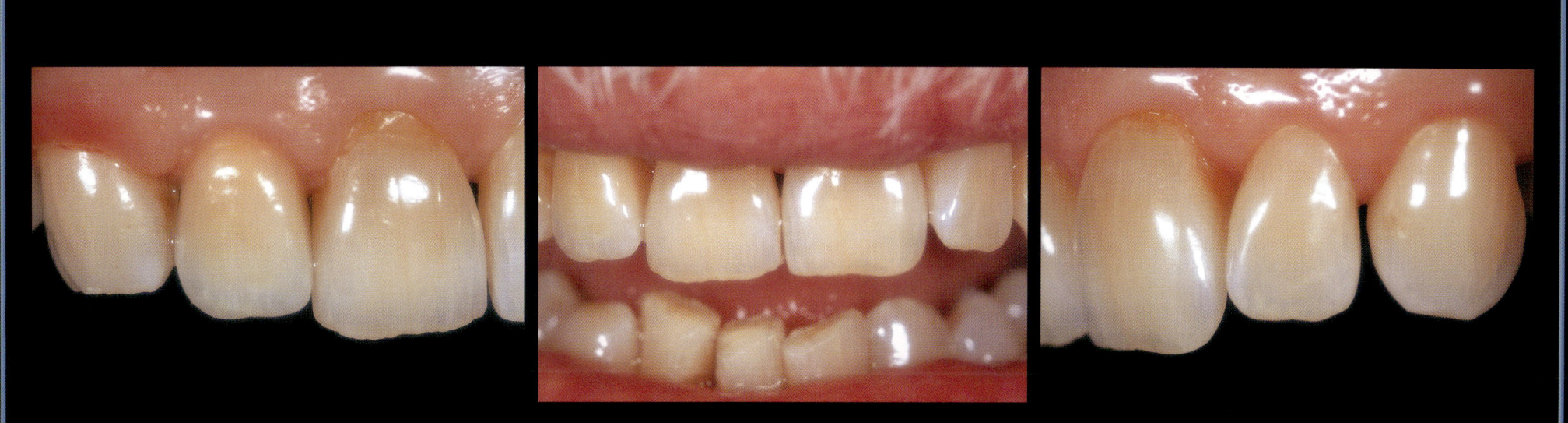

CASE 10

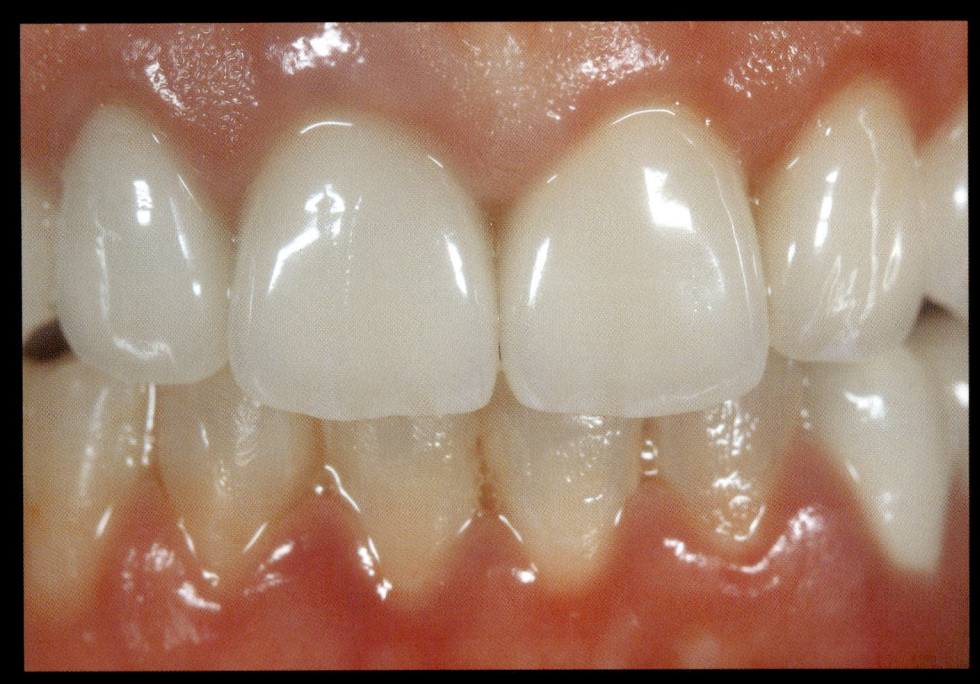

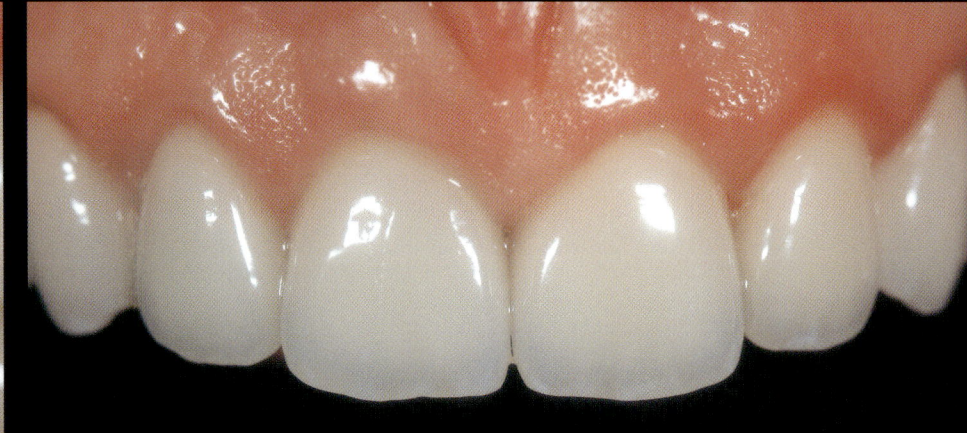

CASE 11

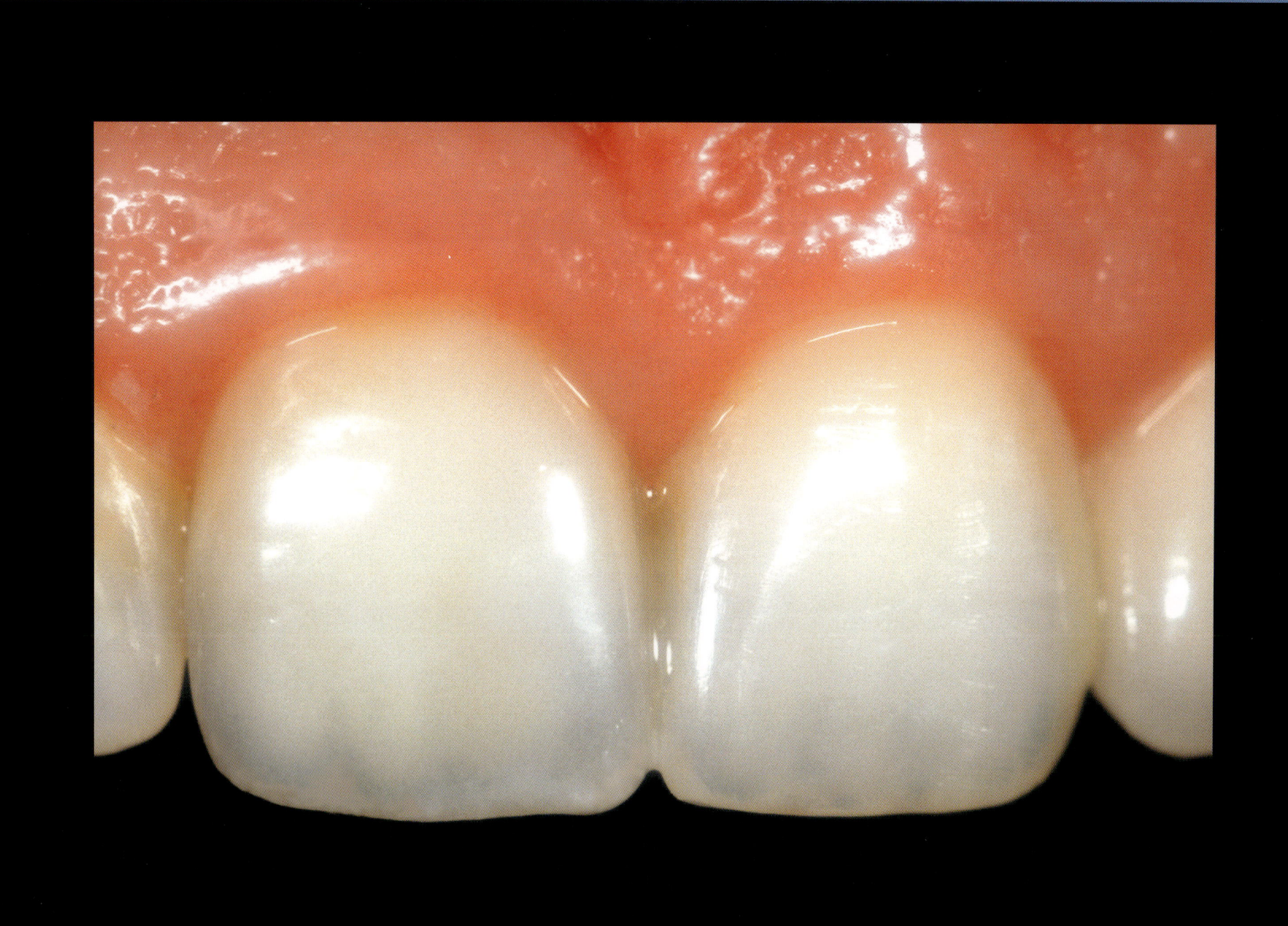

50

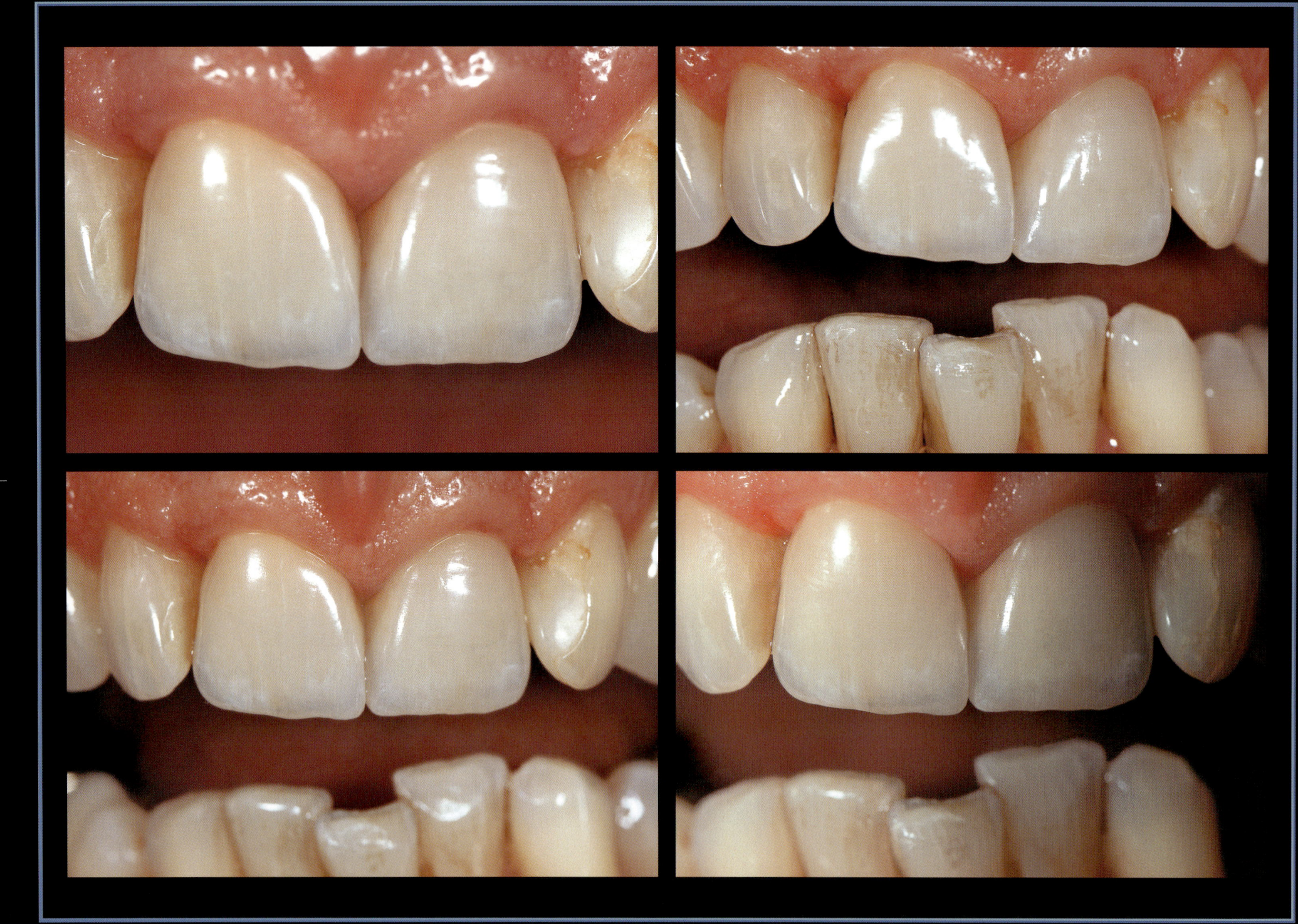

CASE 13

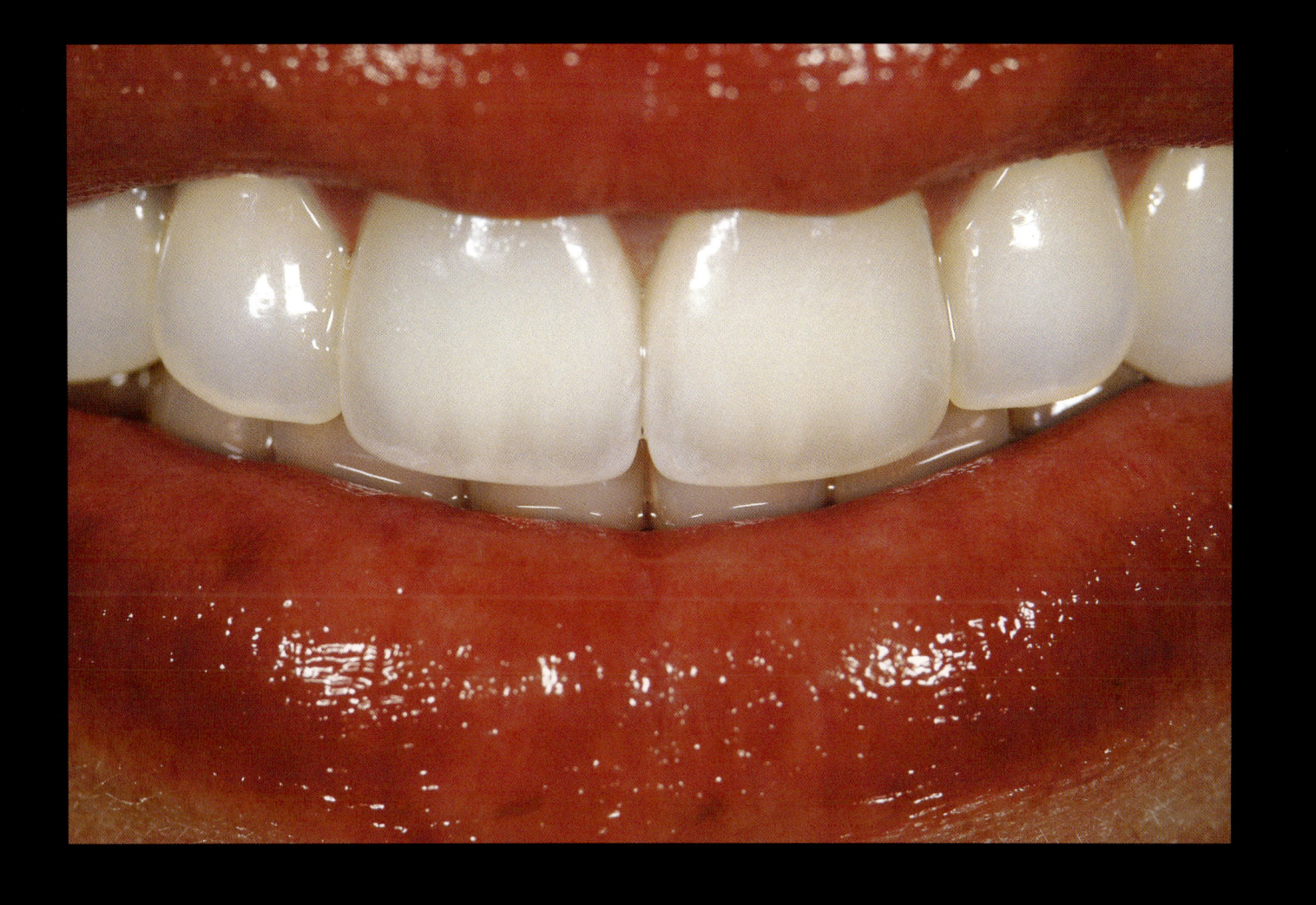

CASE 14

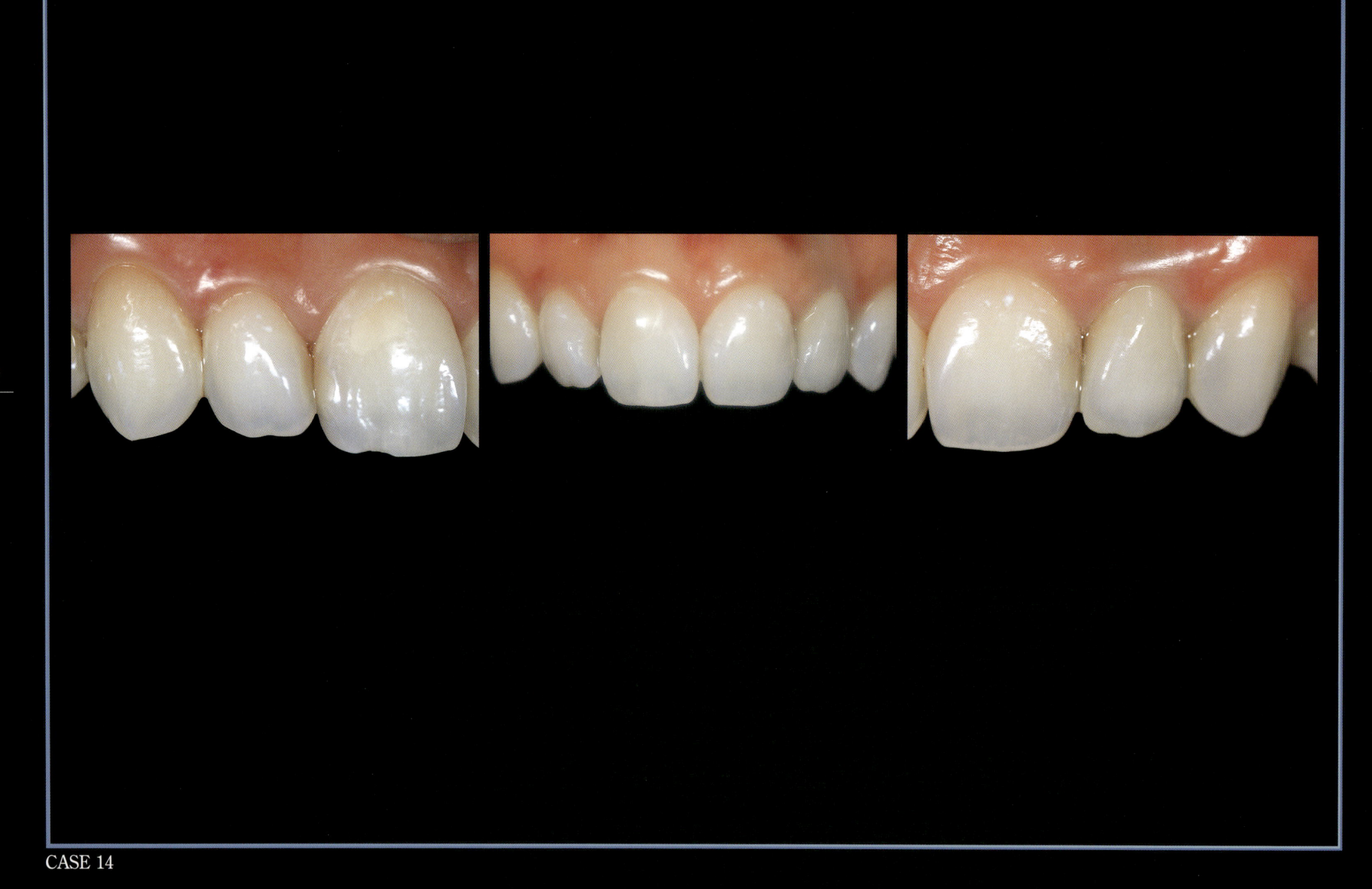

CASE 14

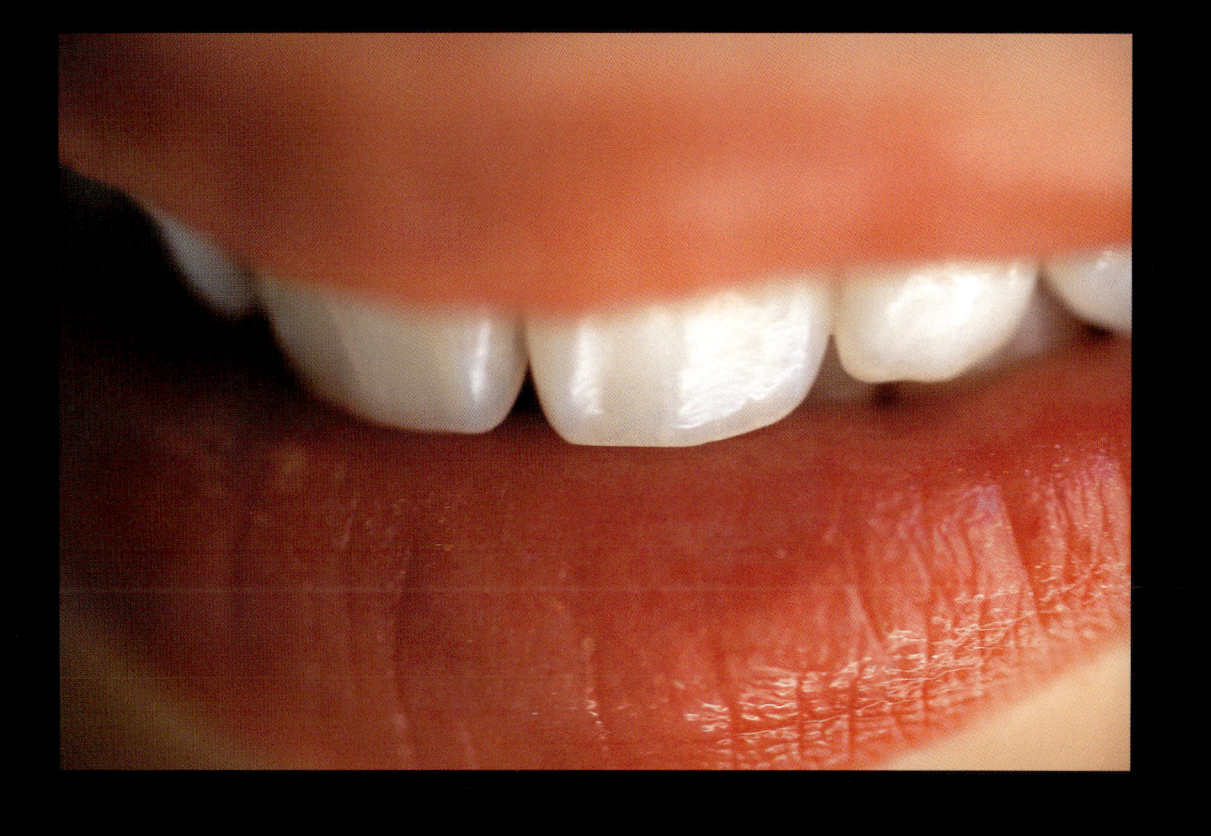

CASE 15

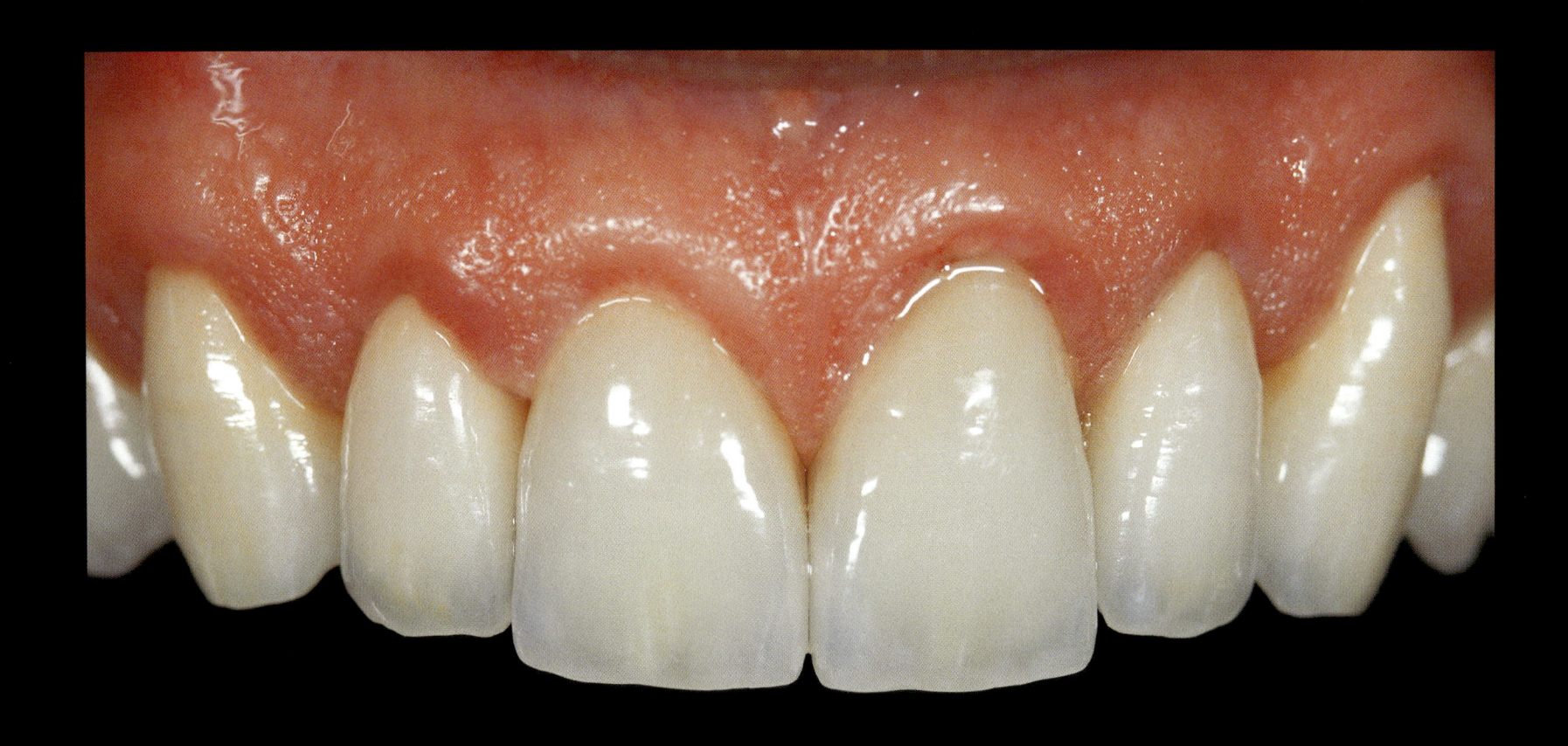

55

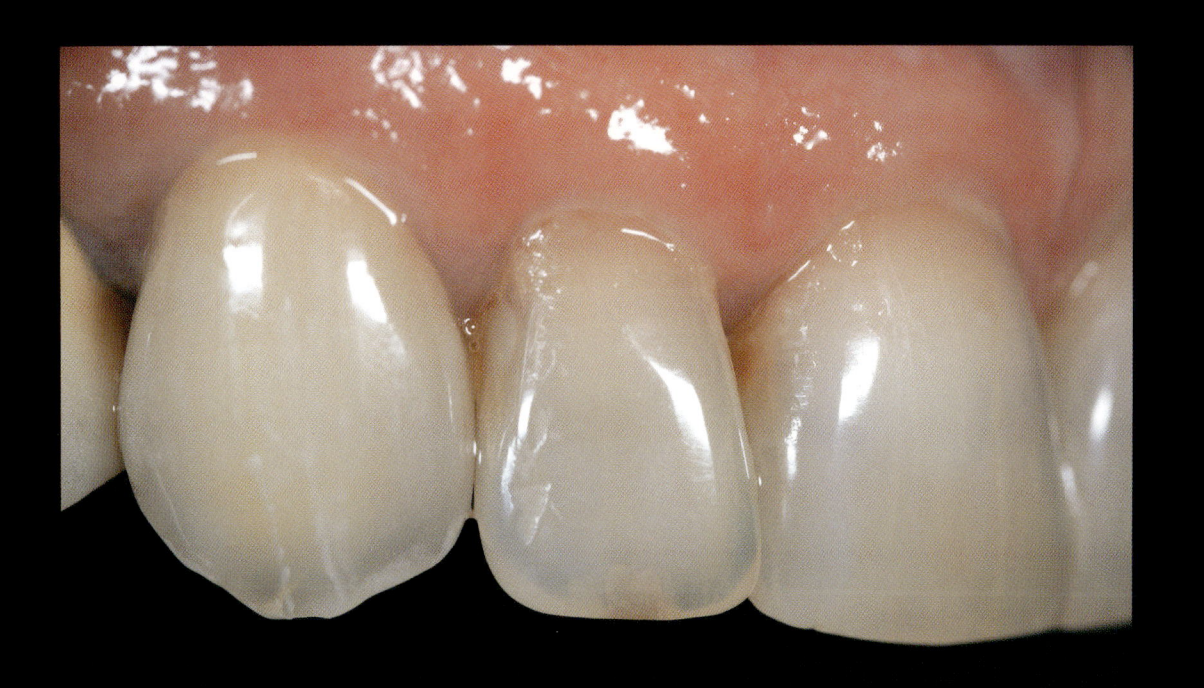

CASE 16

CASE 17

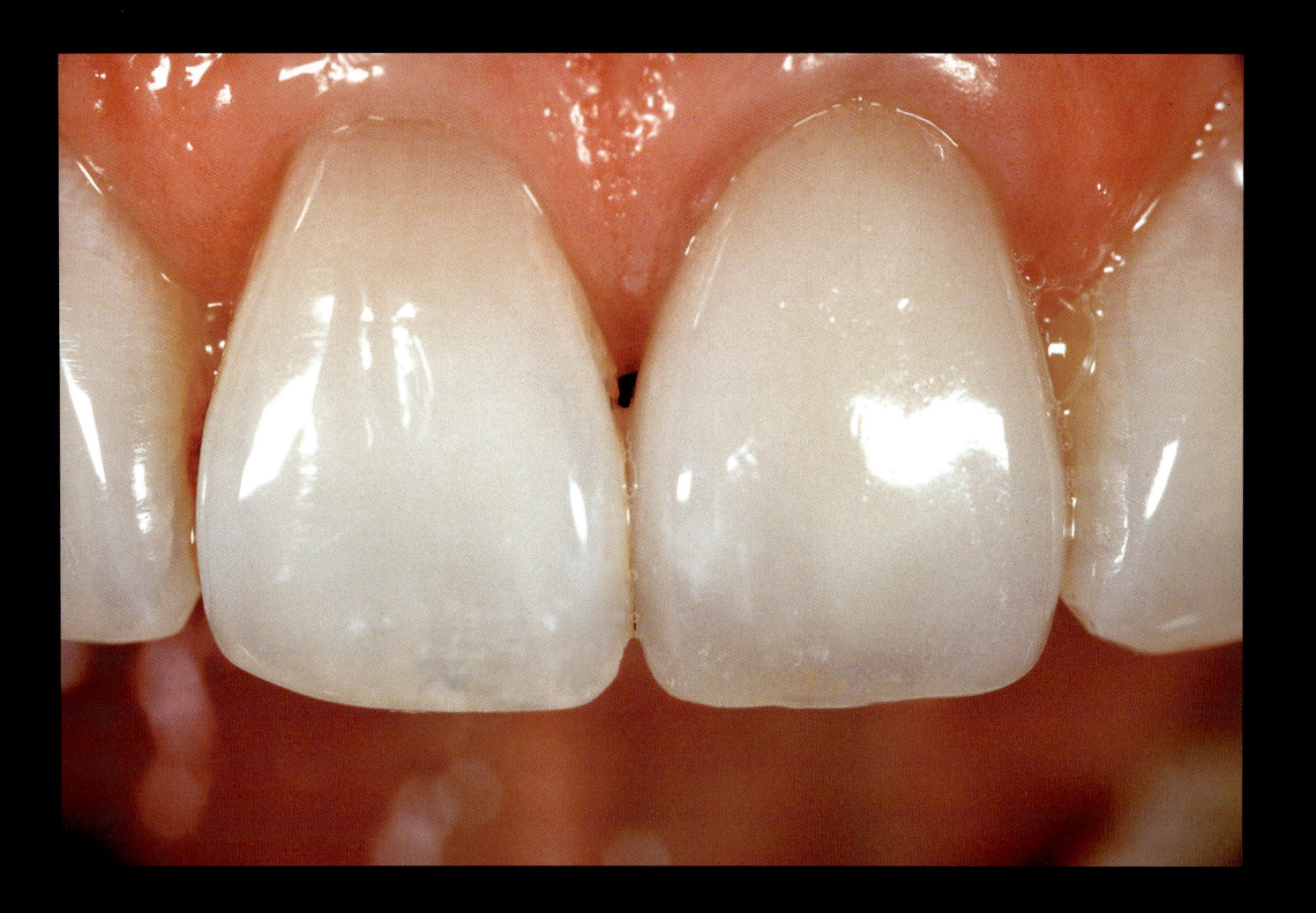

CASE 17

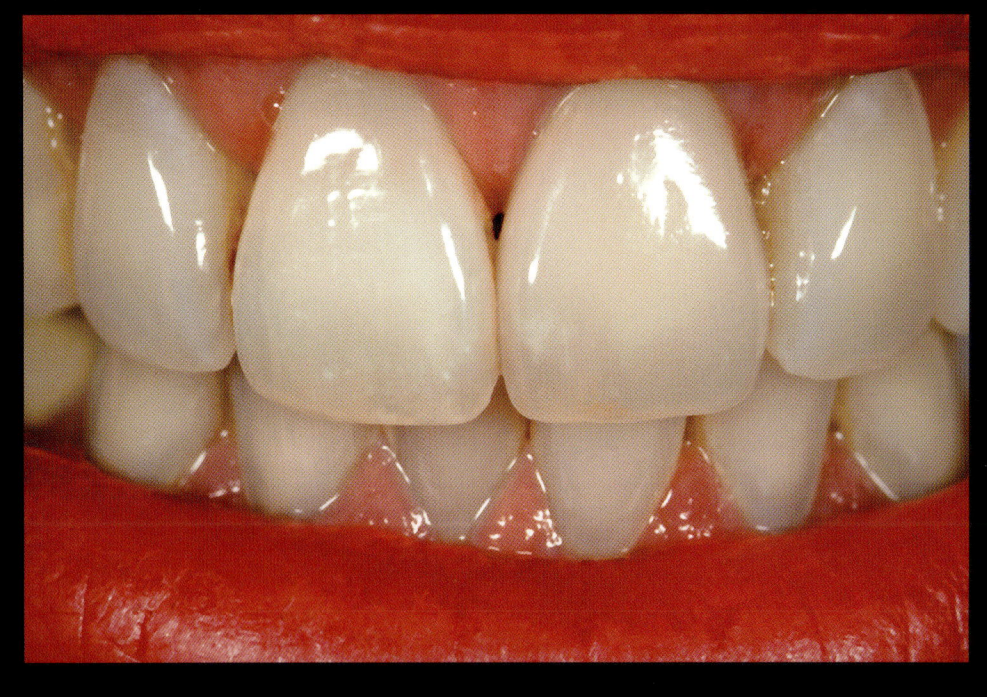

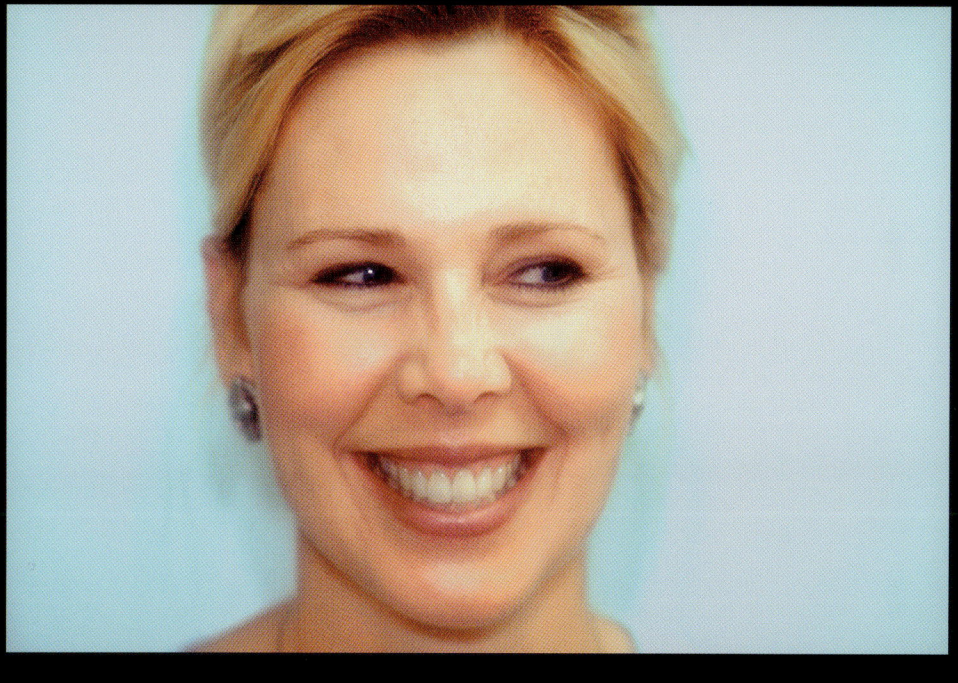

CASE 18

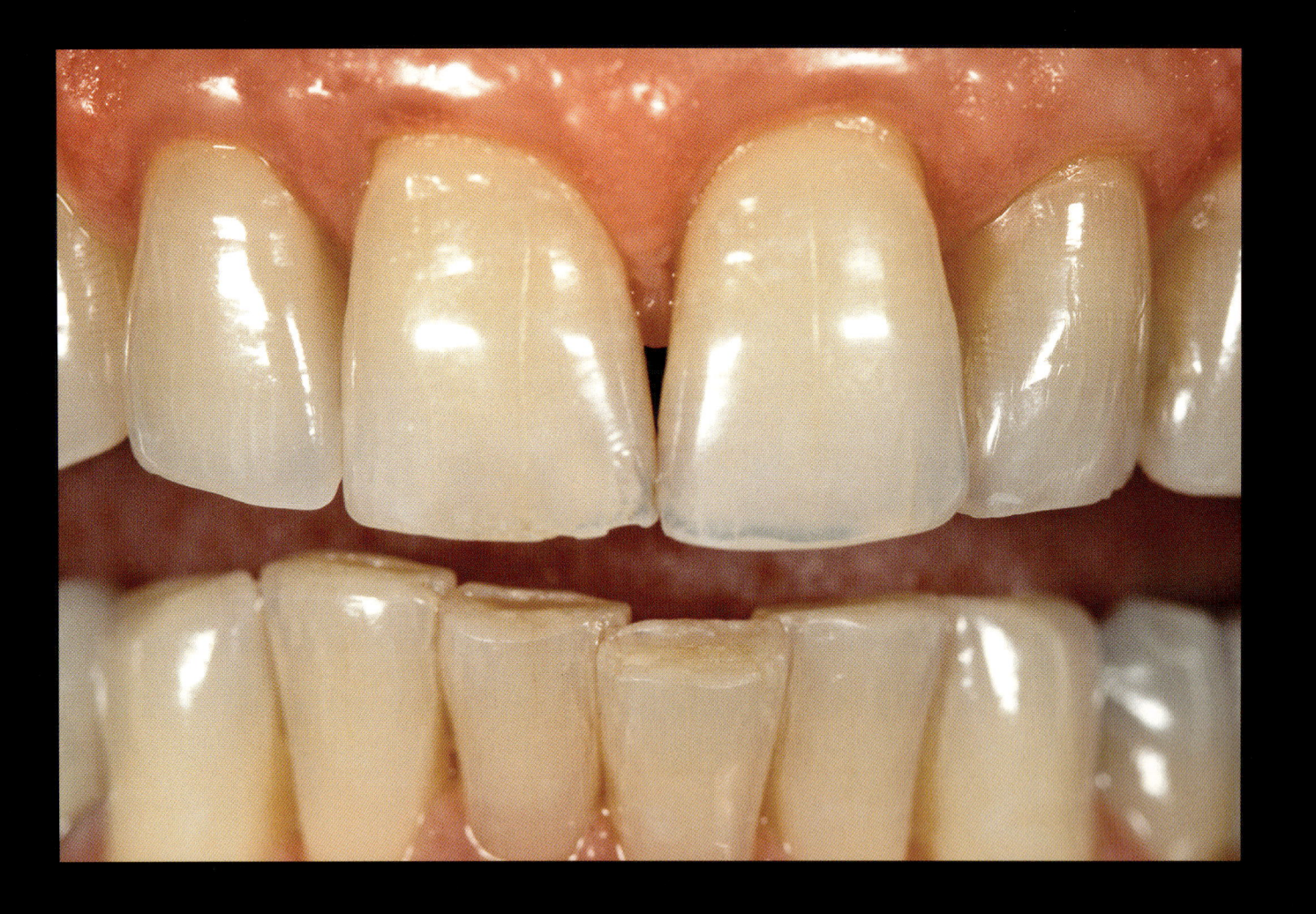

CASE 19

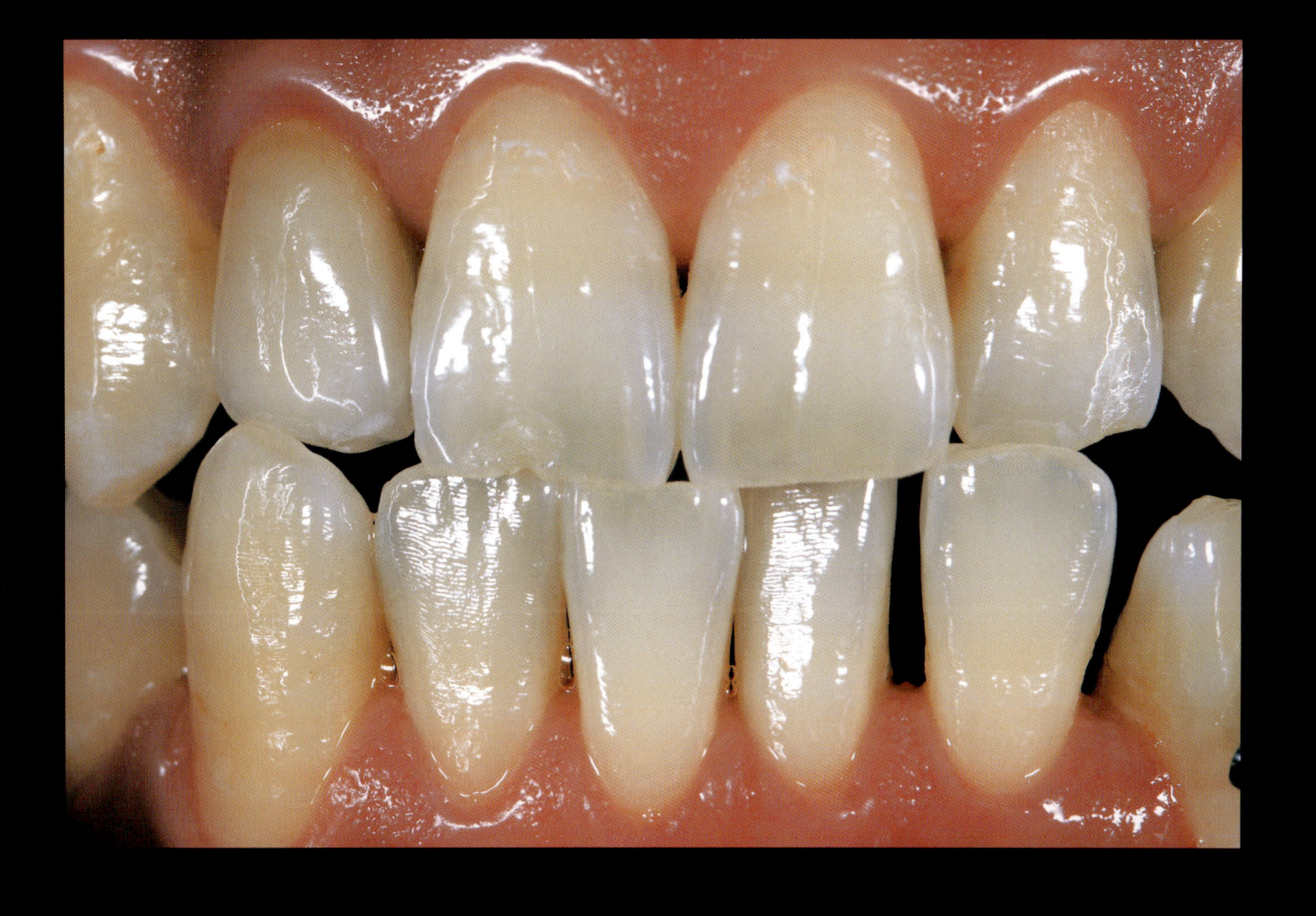

60

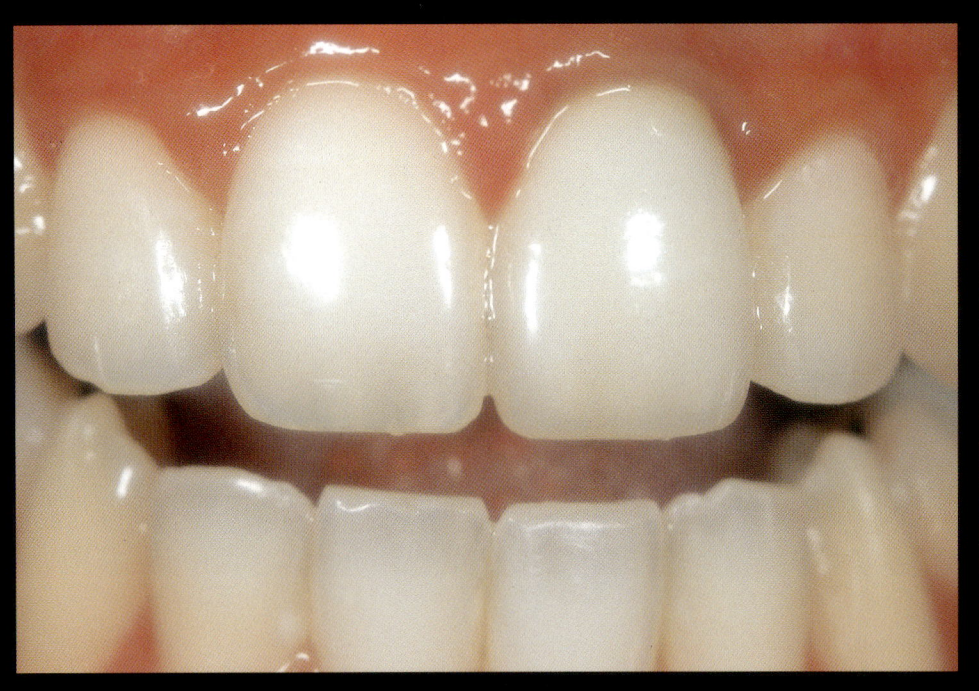

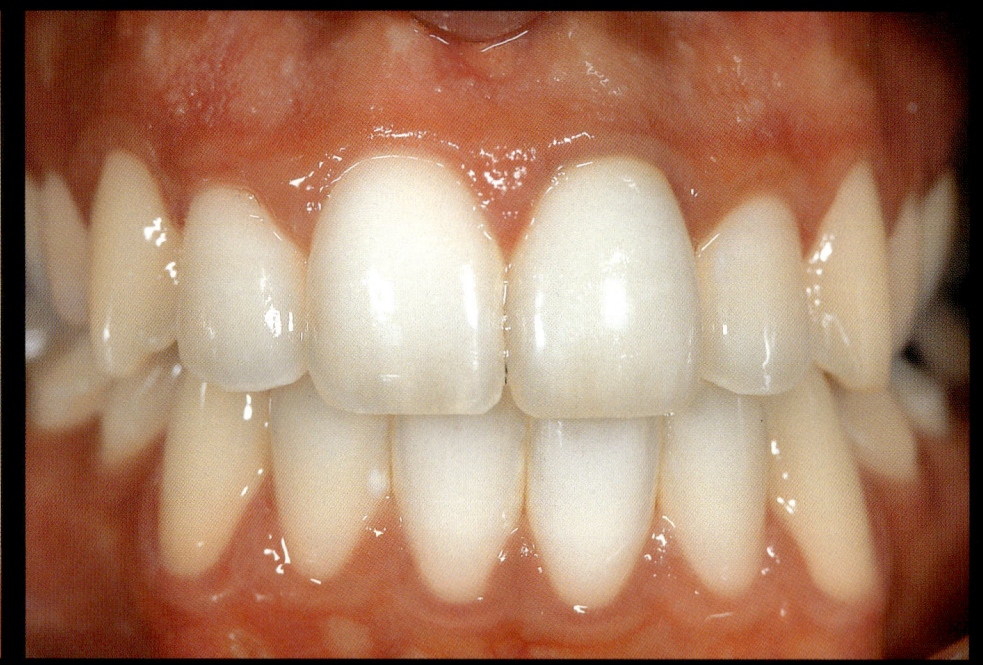

CASE 21

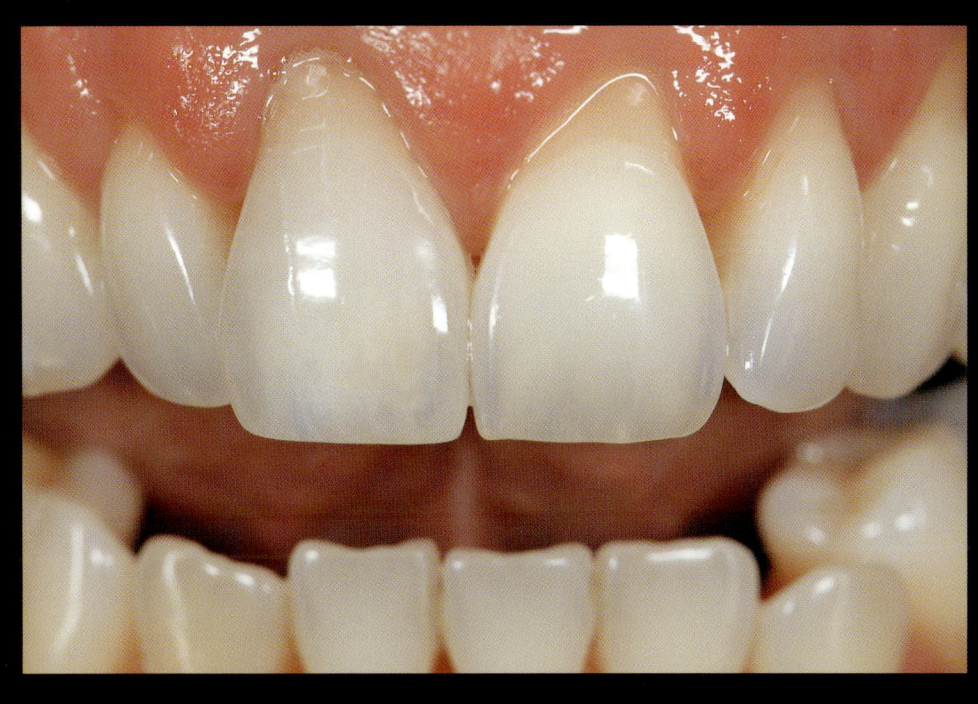

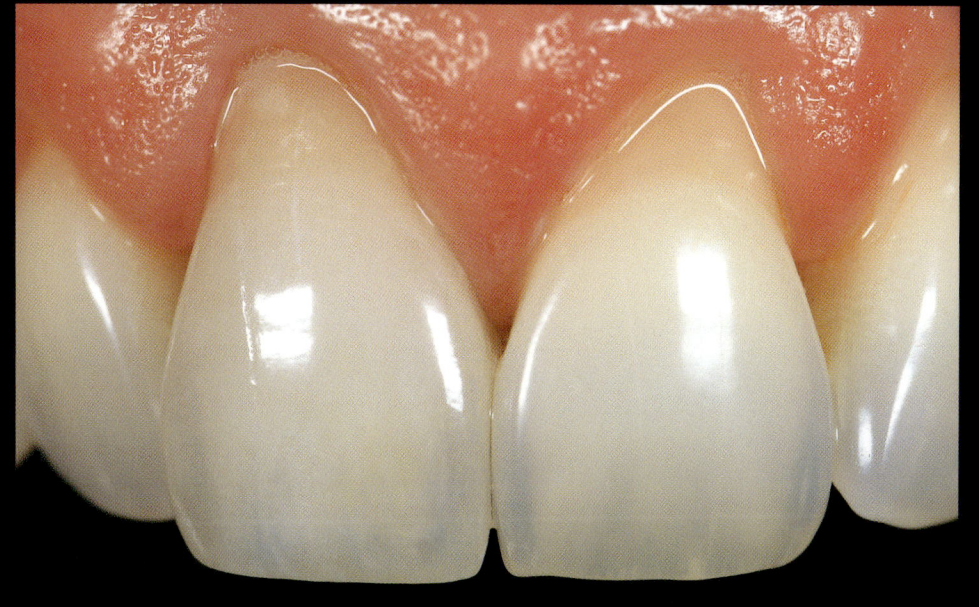

CASE 22

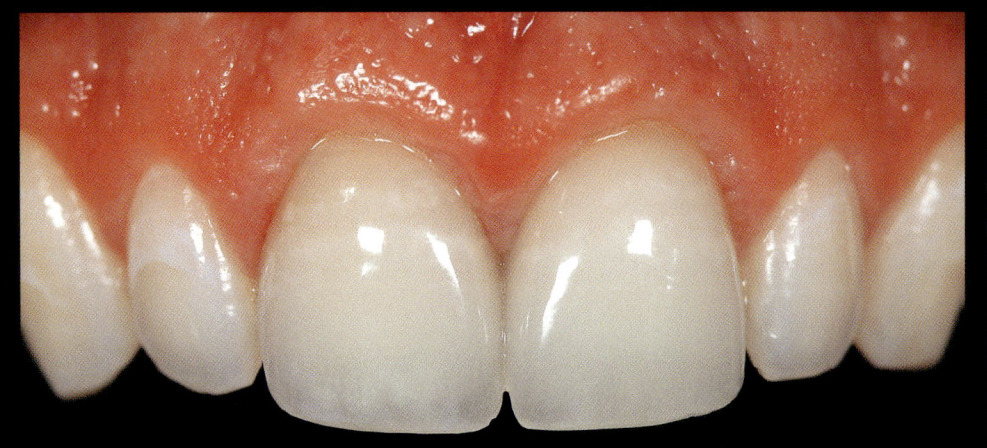

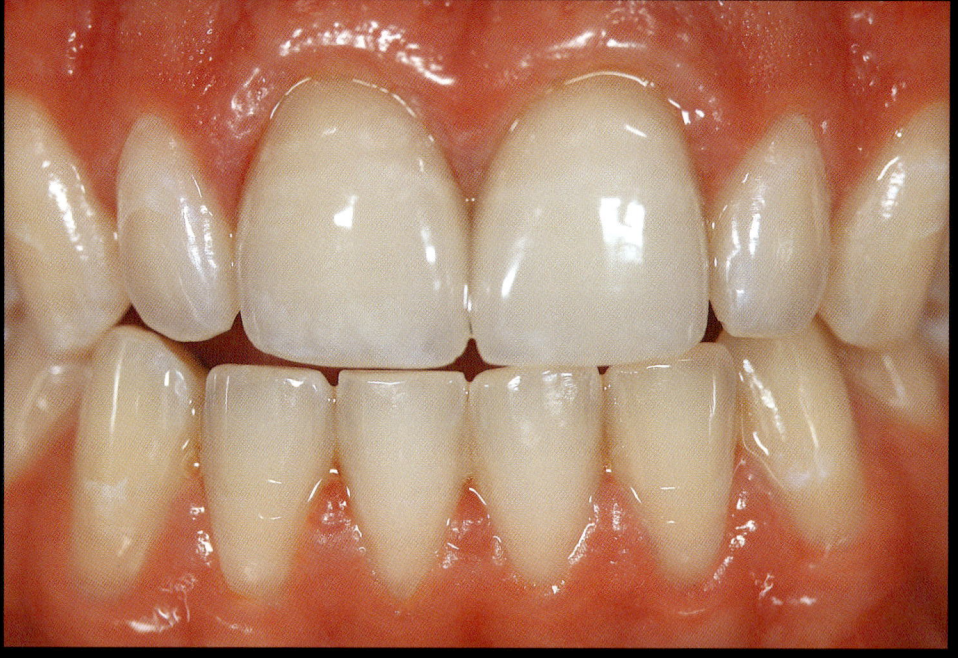

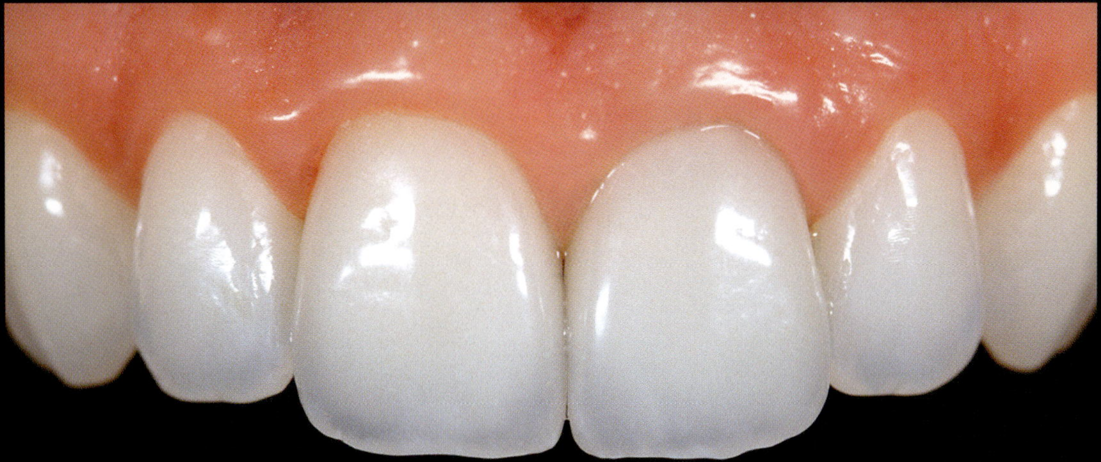

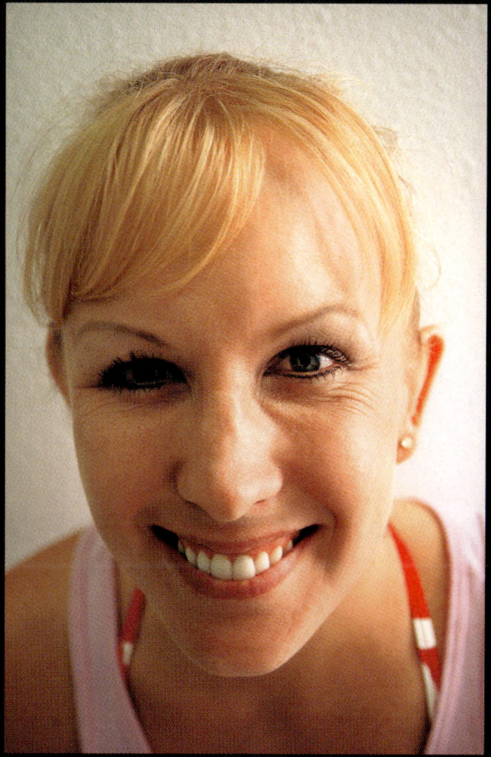

CASE 24

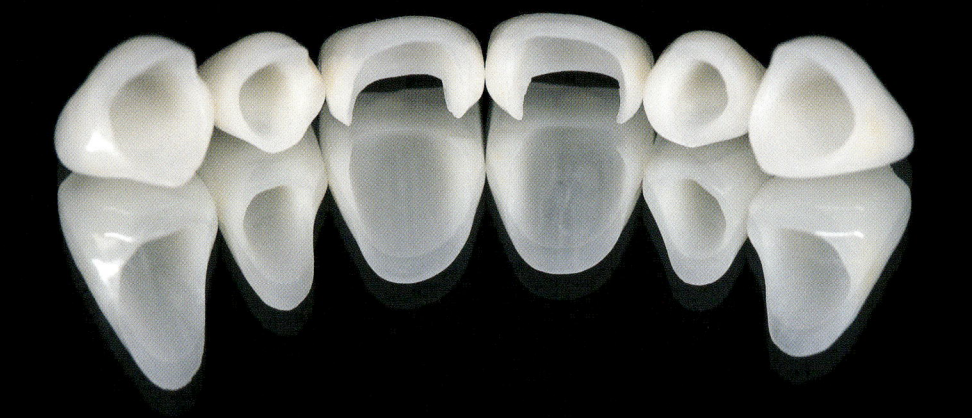

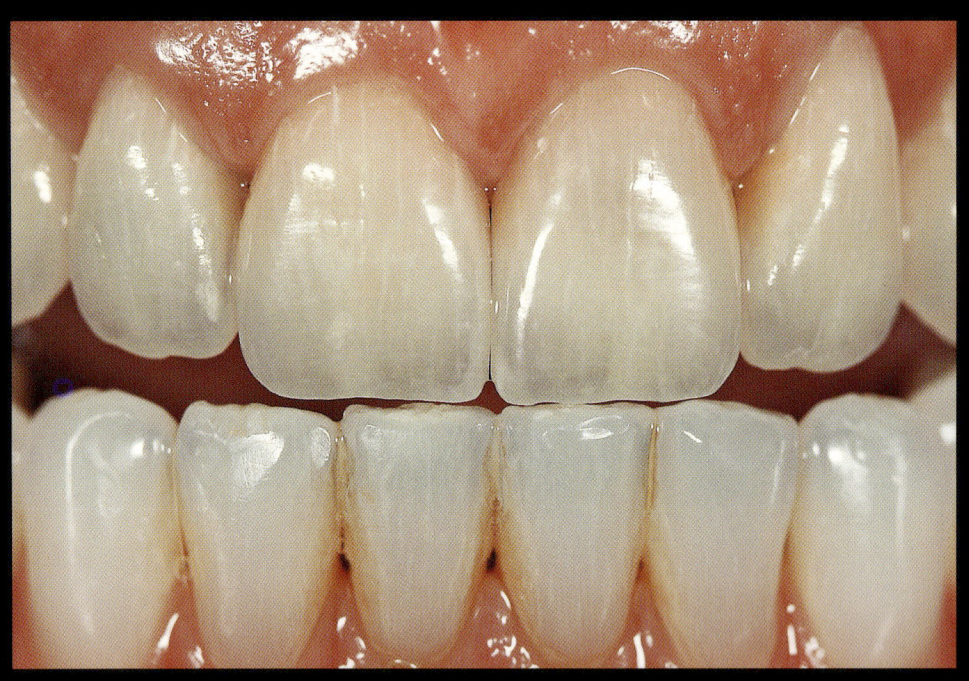

65

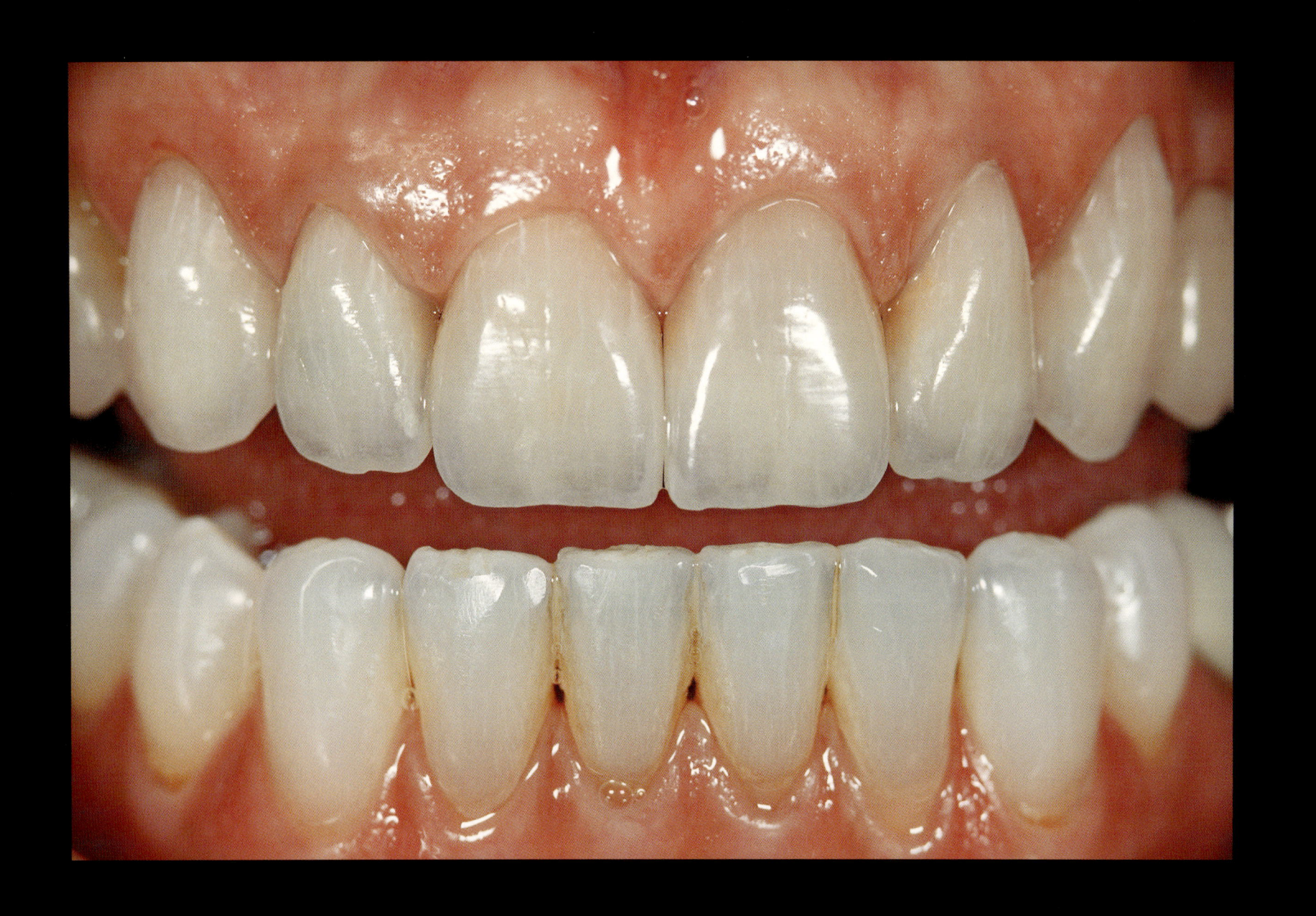

CASE 25

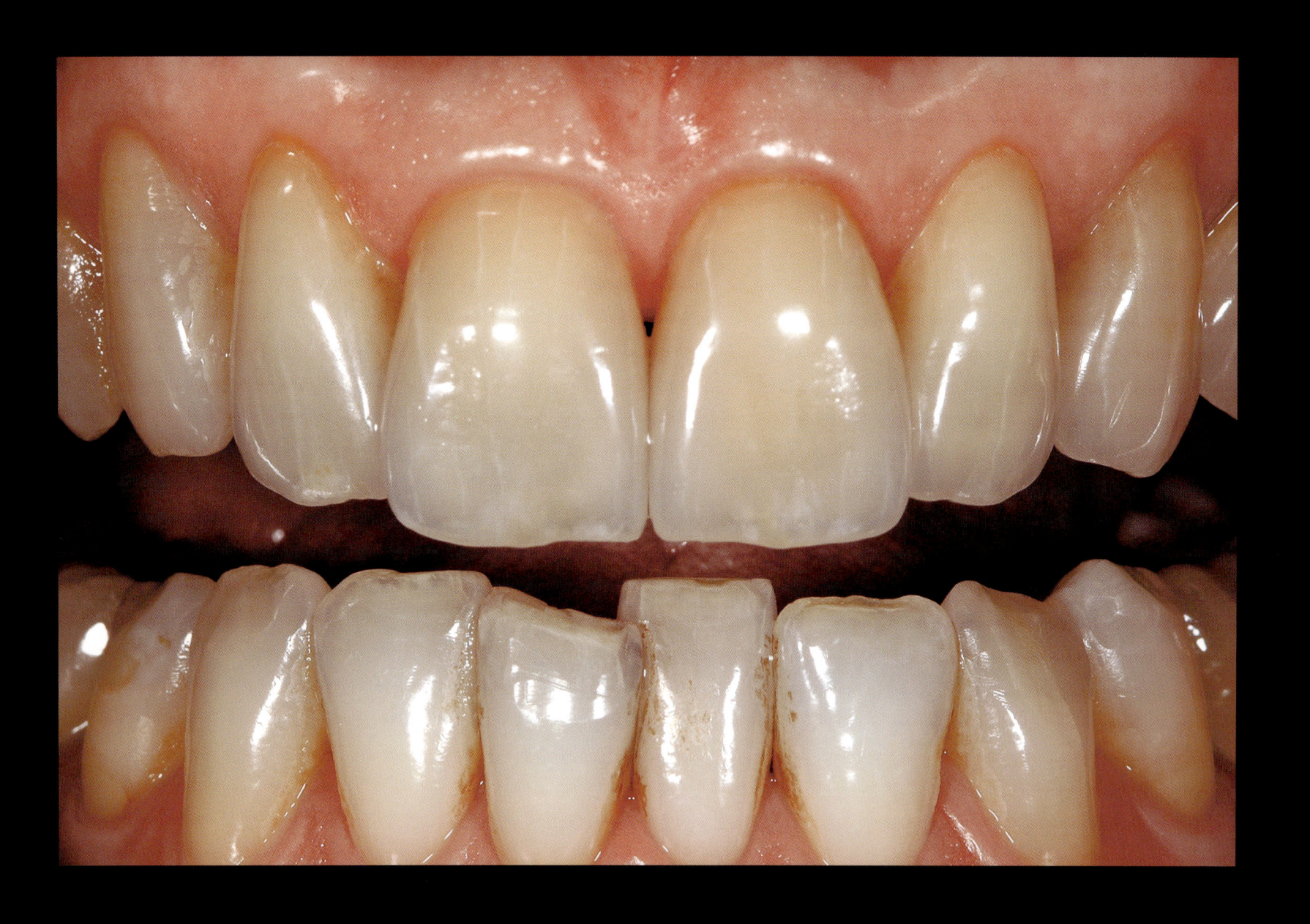

CASE 25

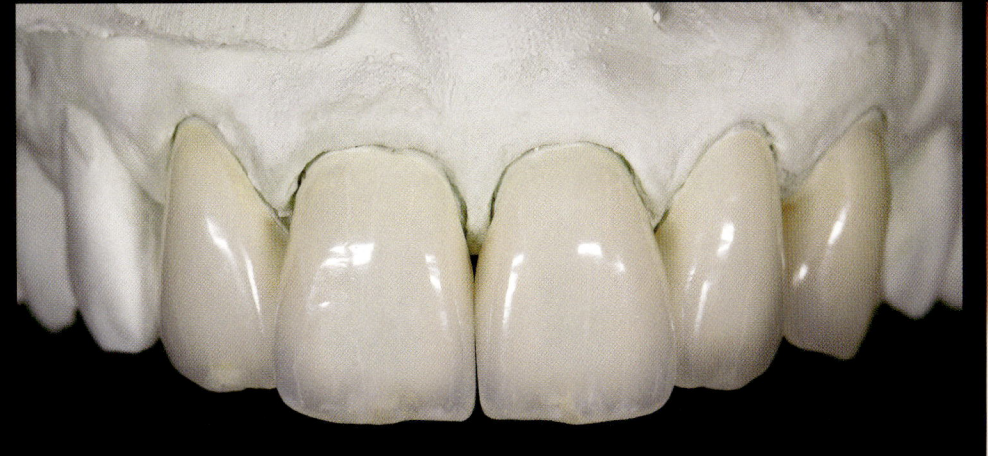

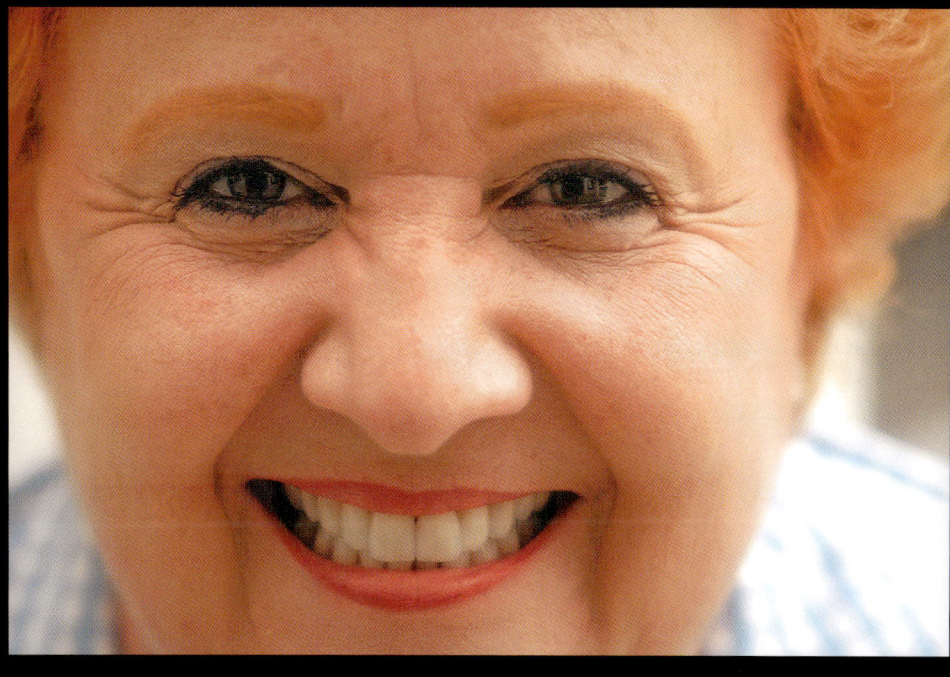

68

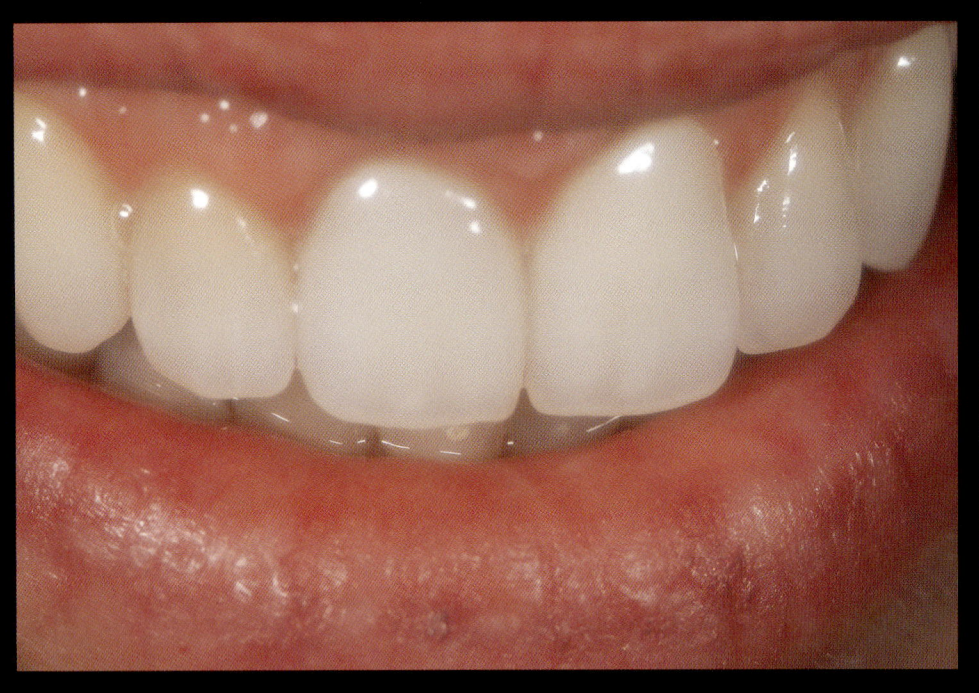

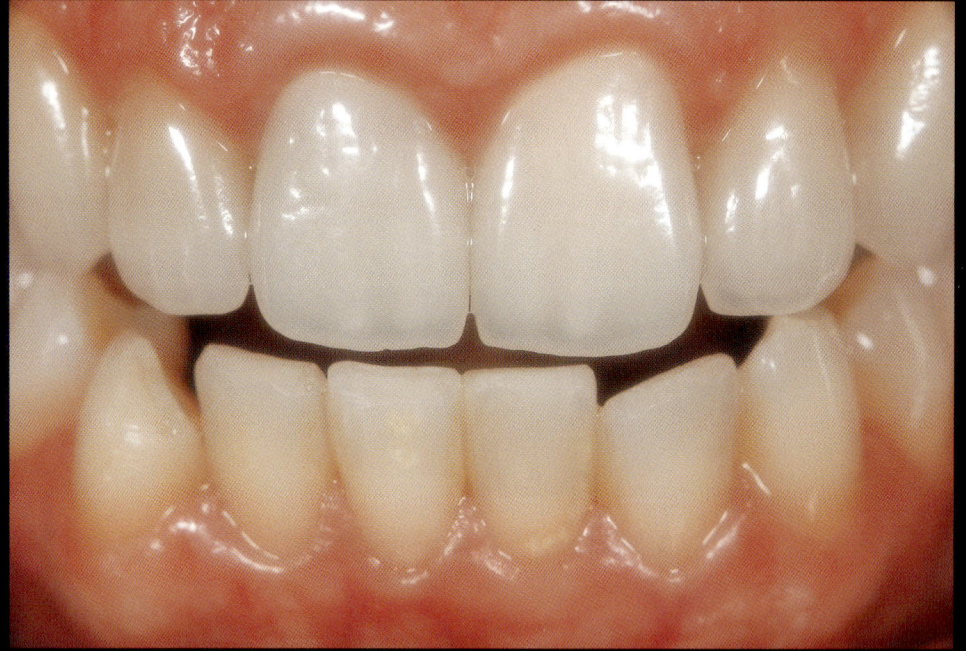

CASE 27

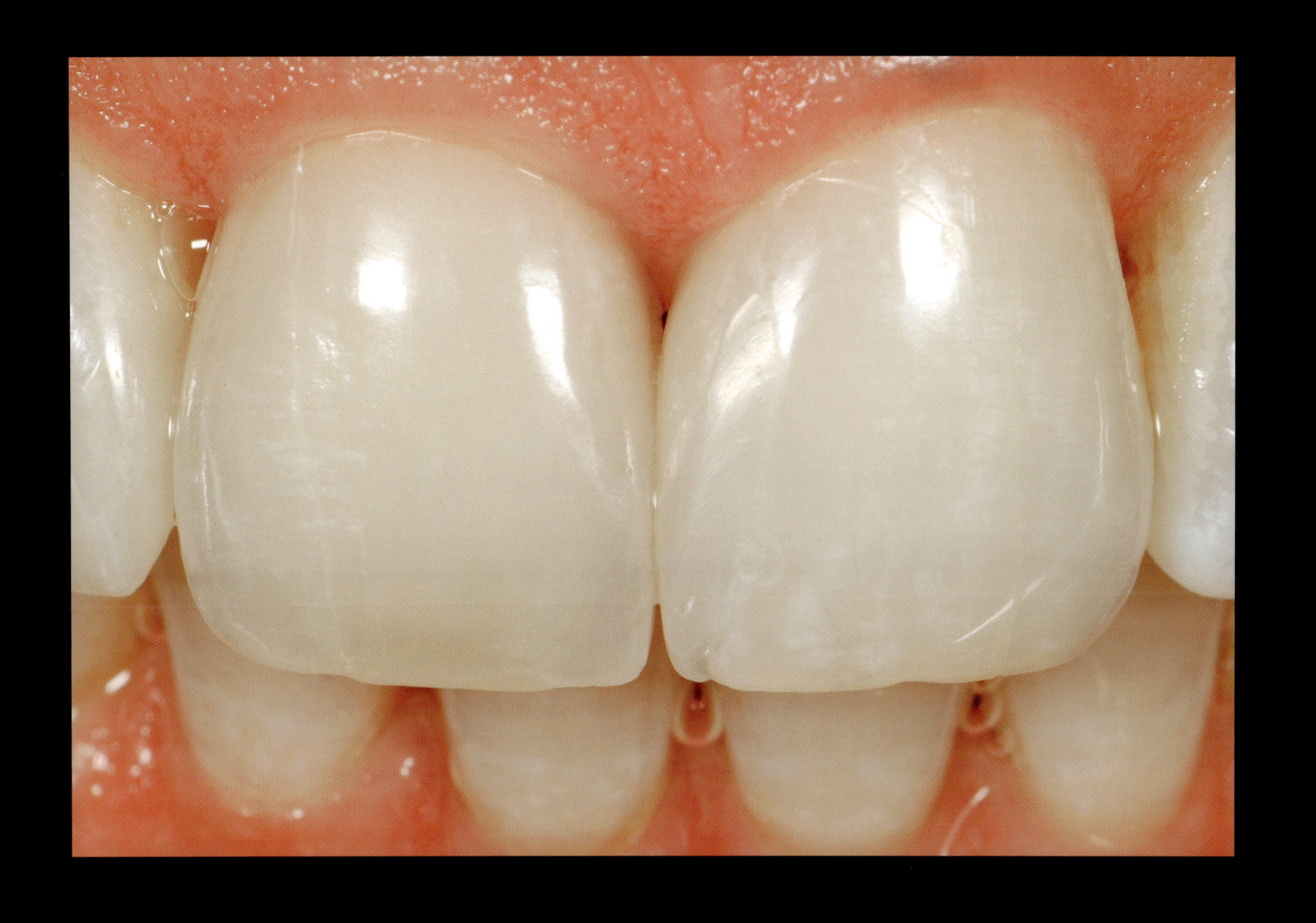

CASE 28

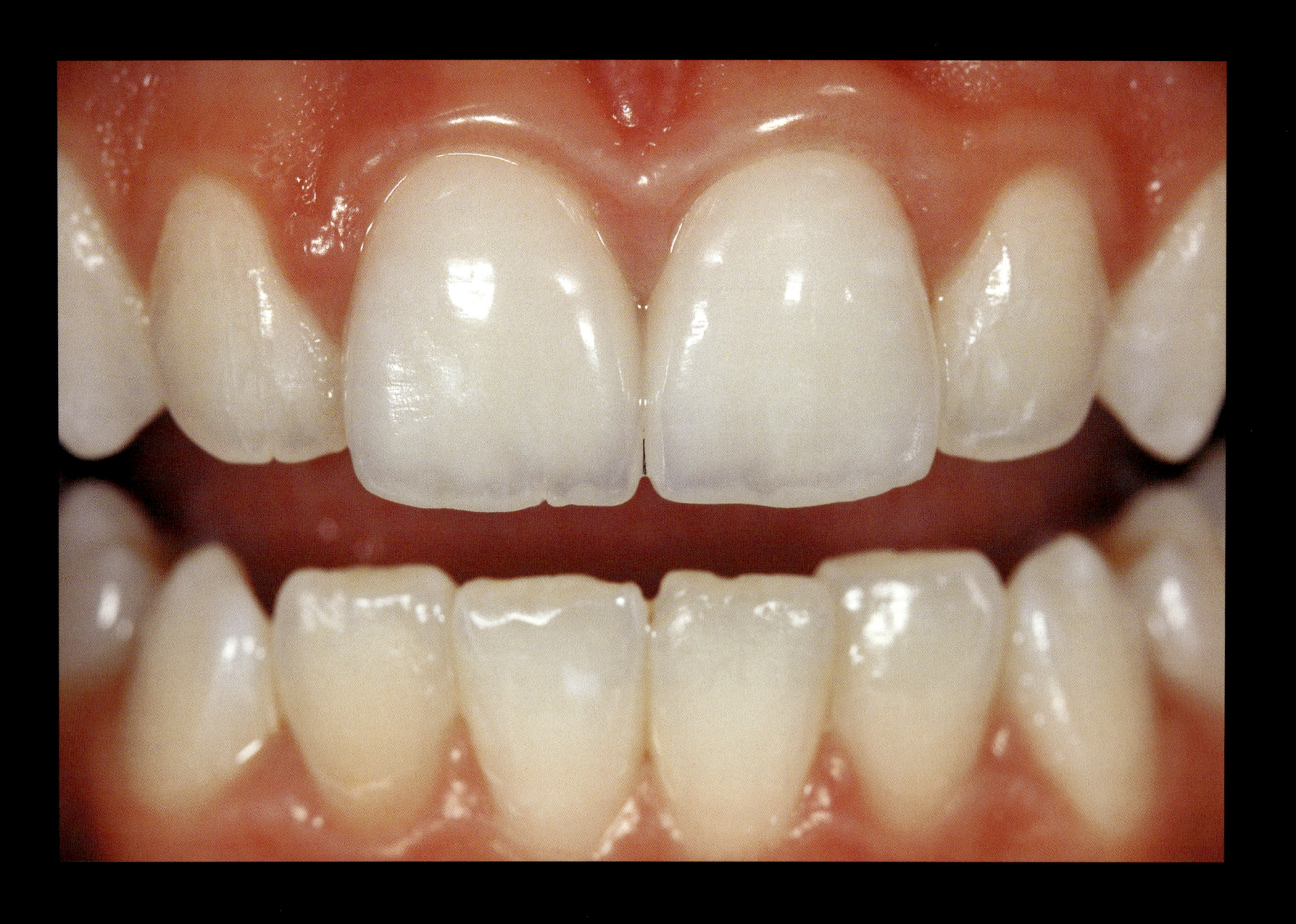

CASE 28

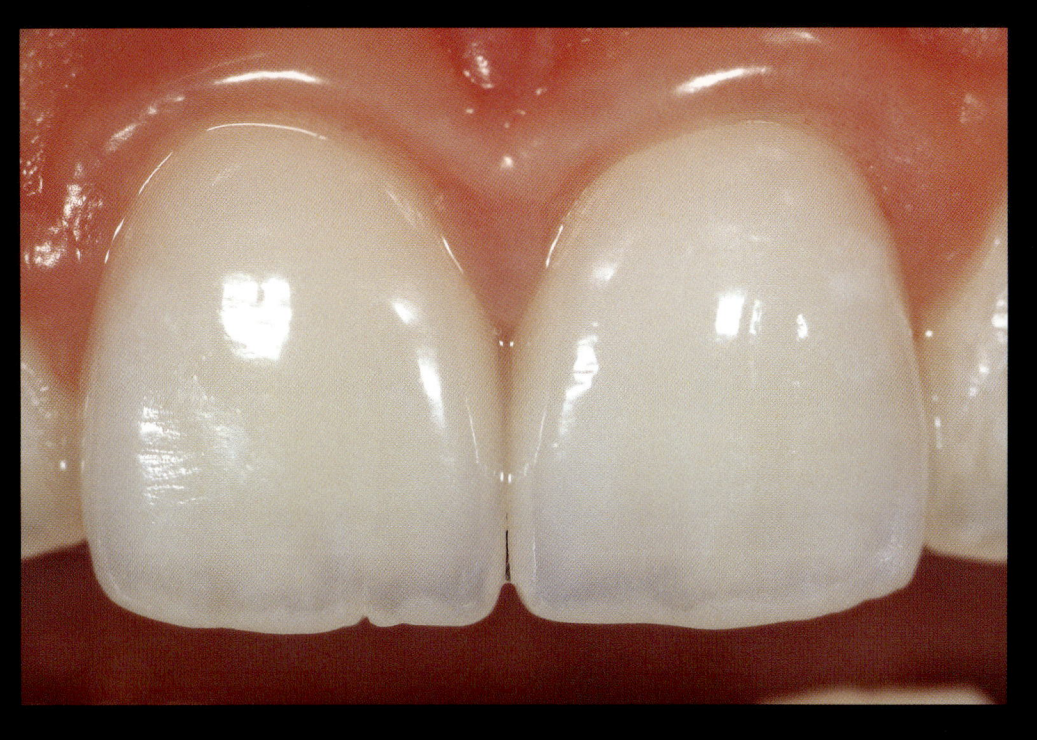

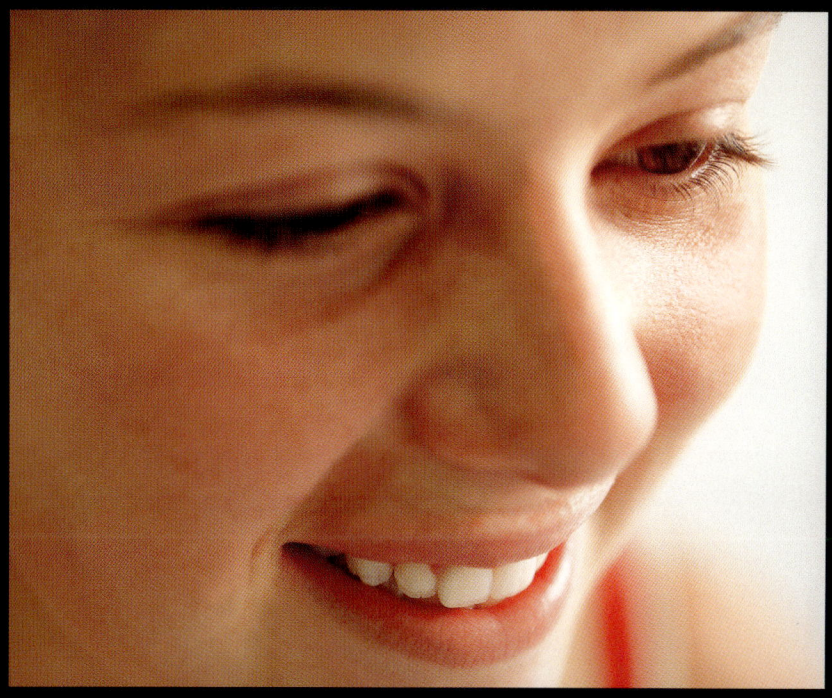

Chapter 3
Porcelain Laminate Veneer

CASE 29

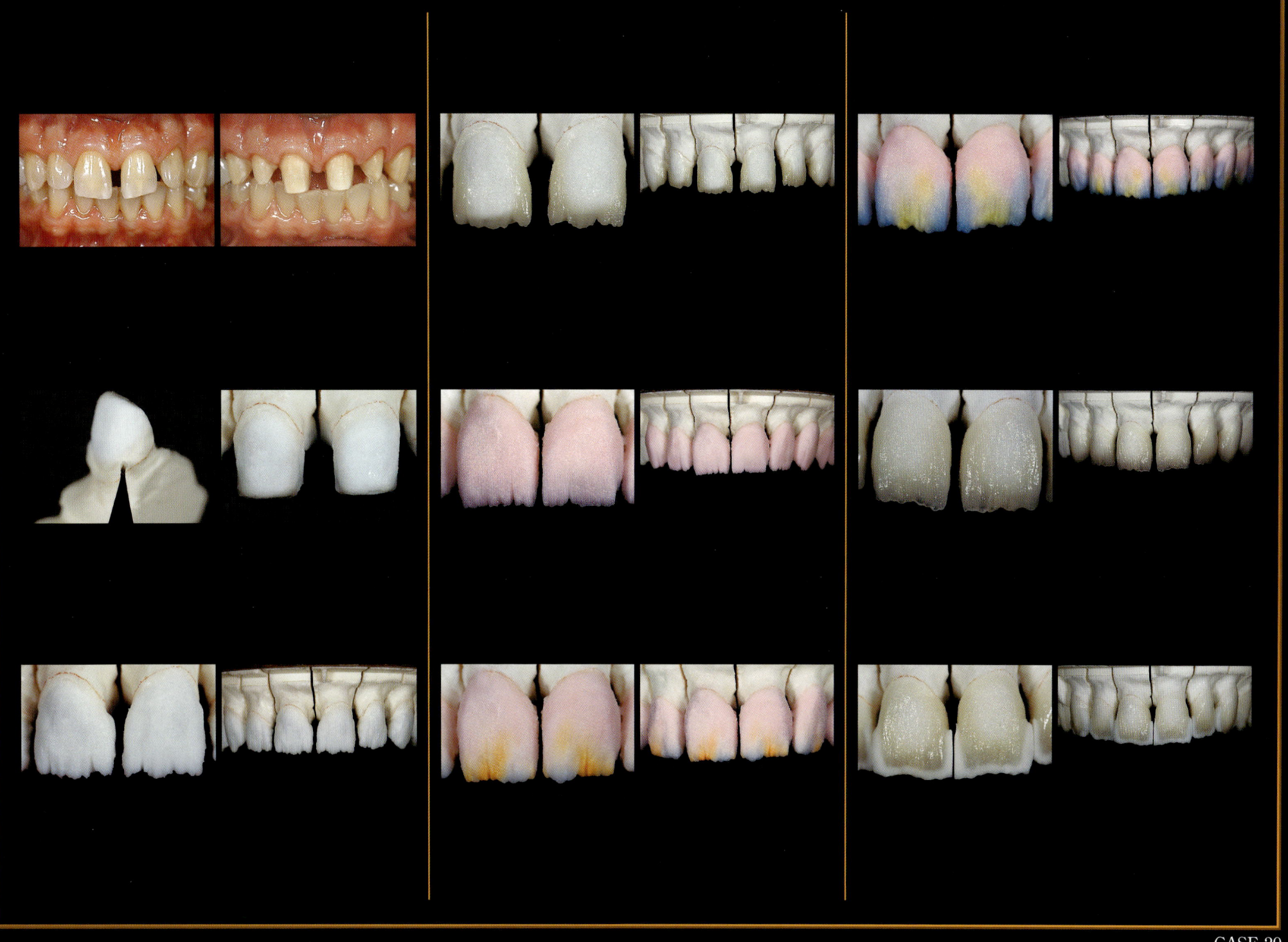

CASE 29

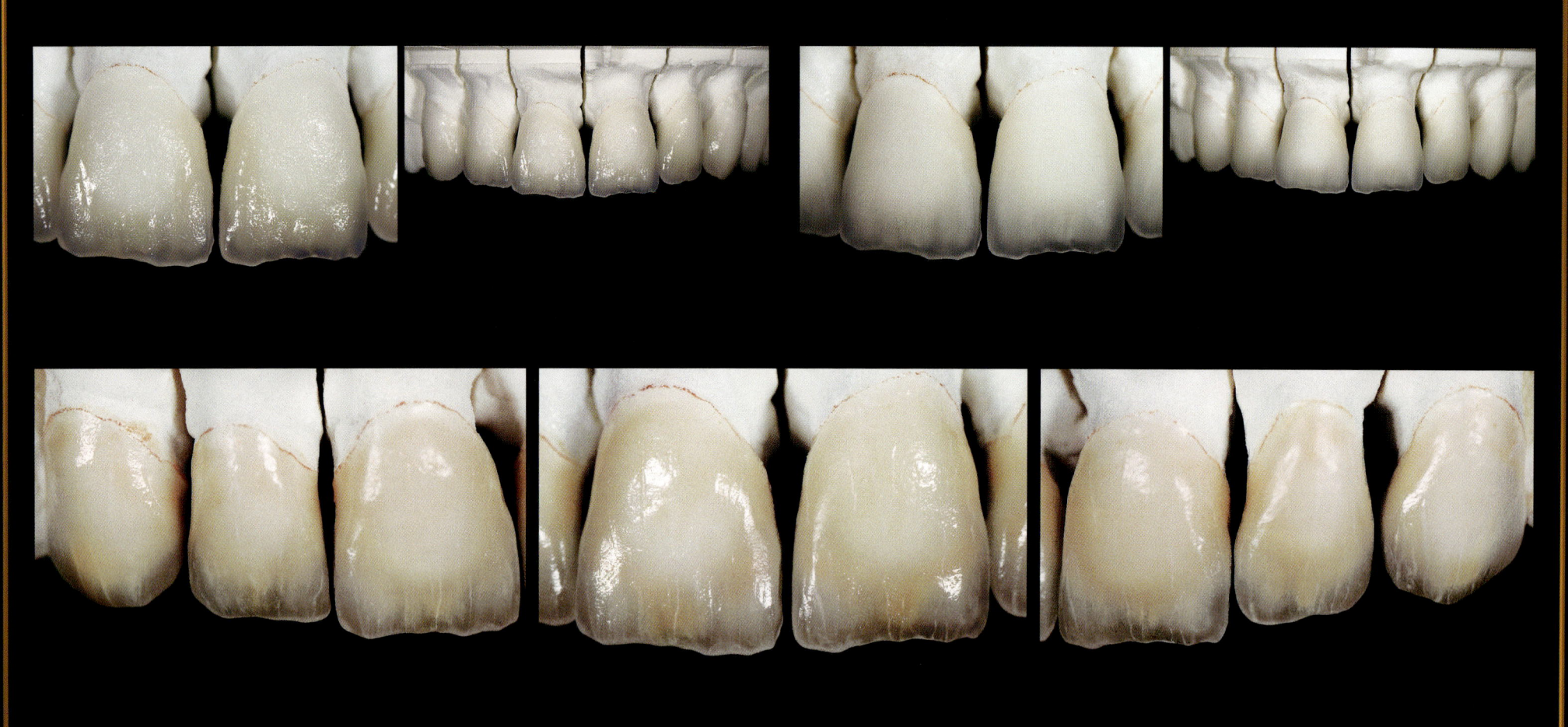

CASE 29

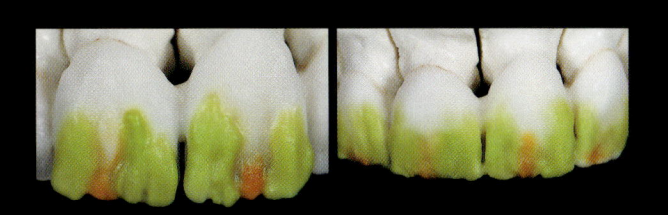

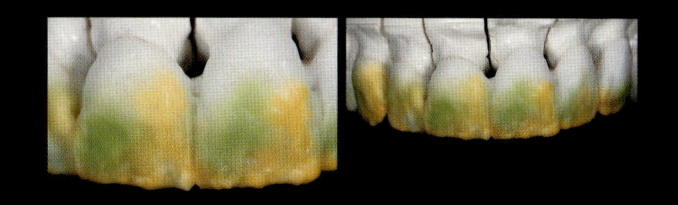

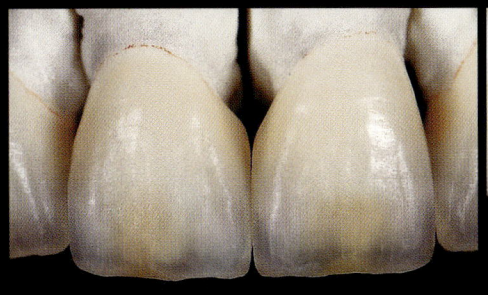

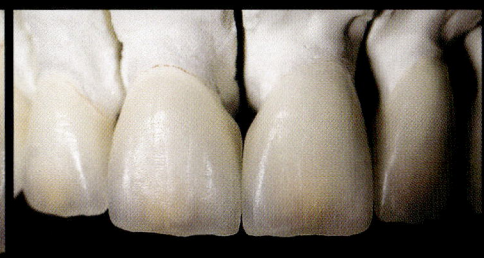

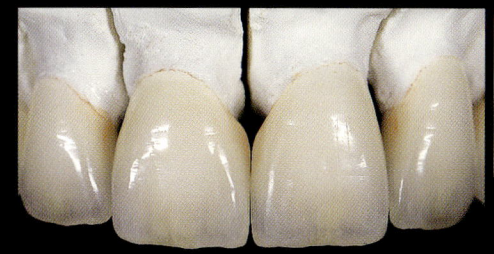

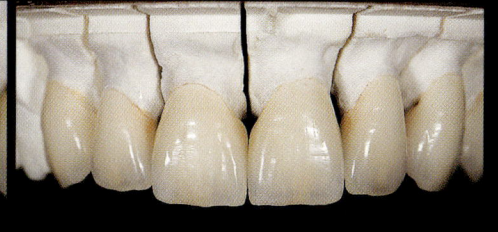

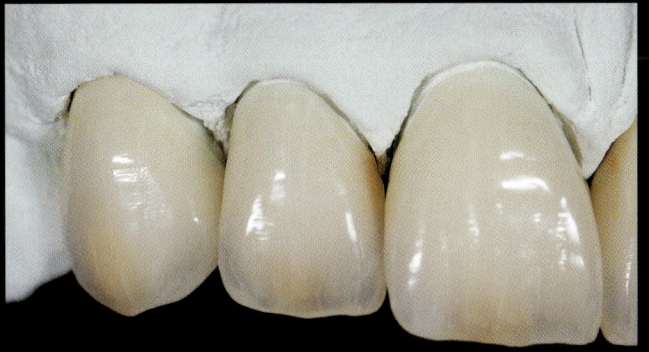

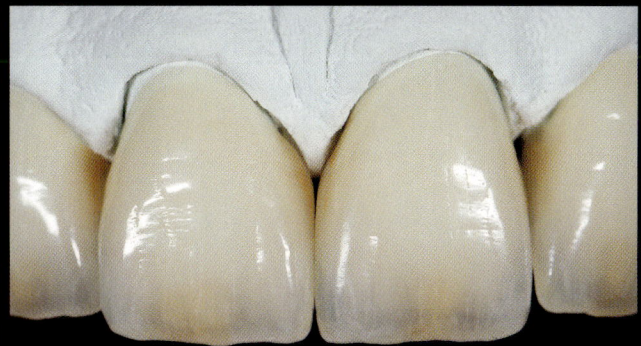

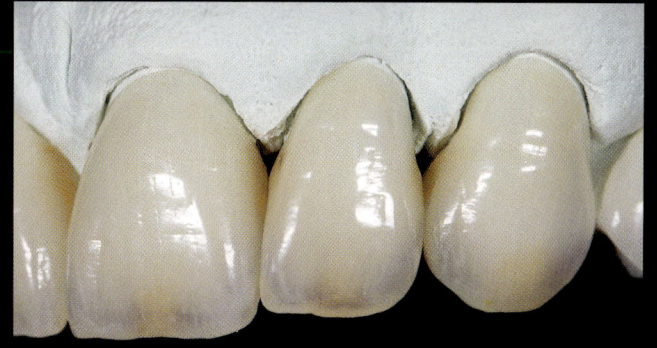

CASE 29

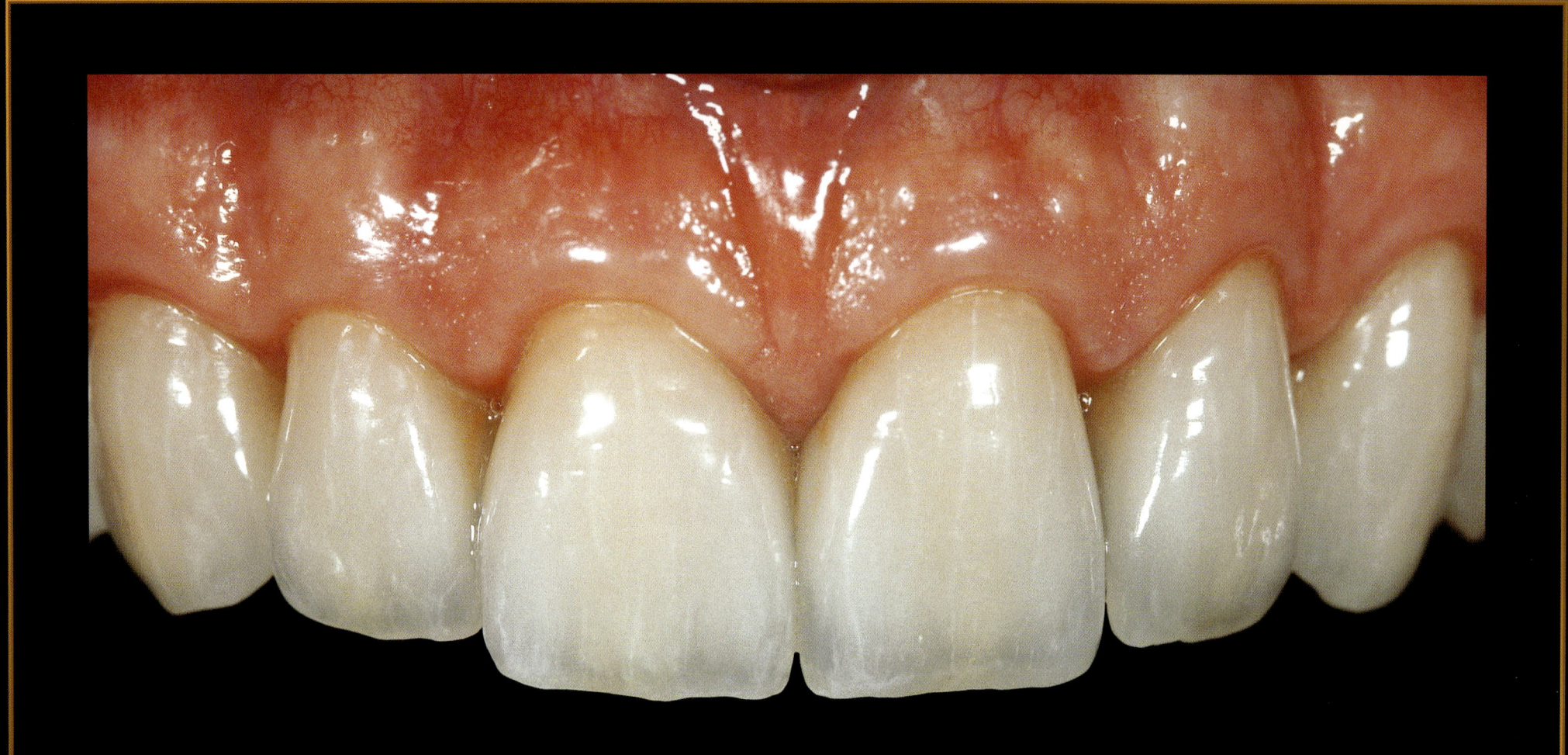

CASE 29

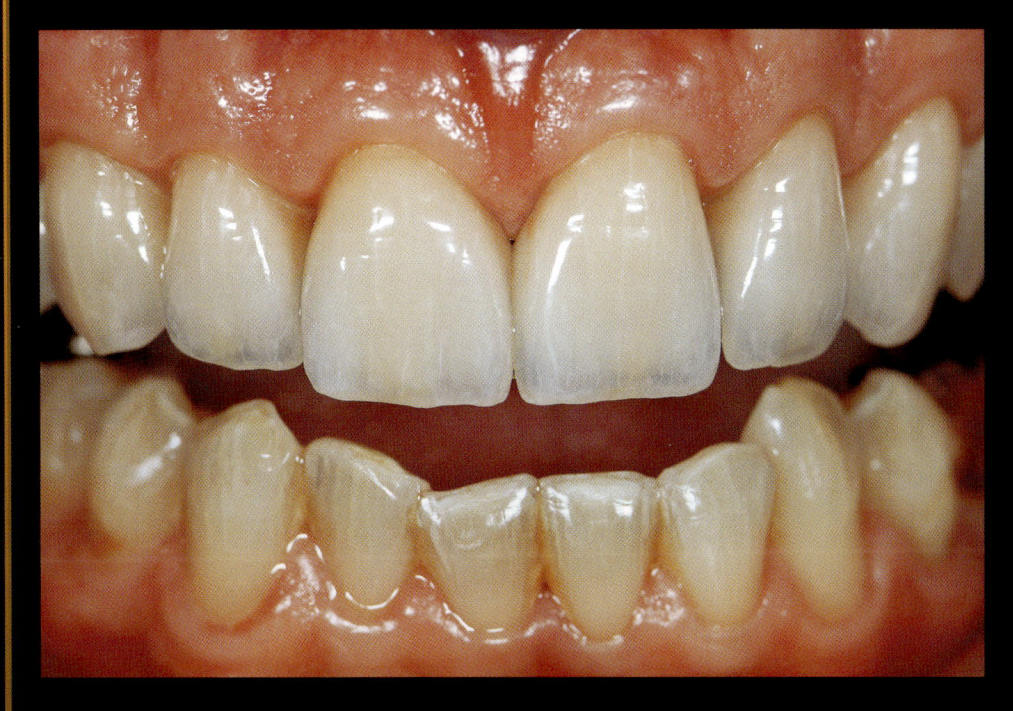

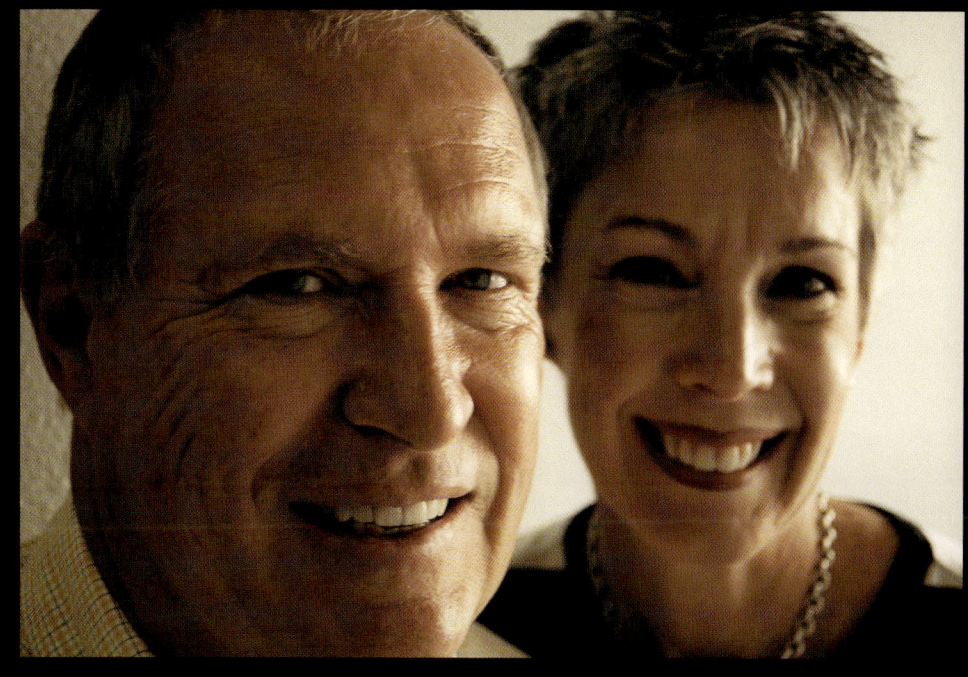

CASE 30

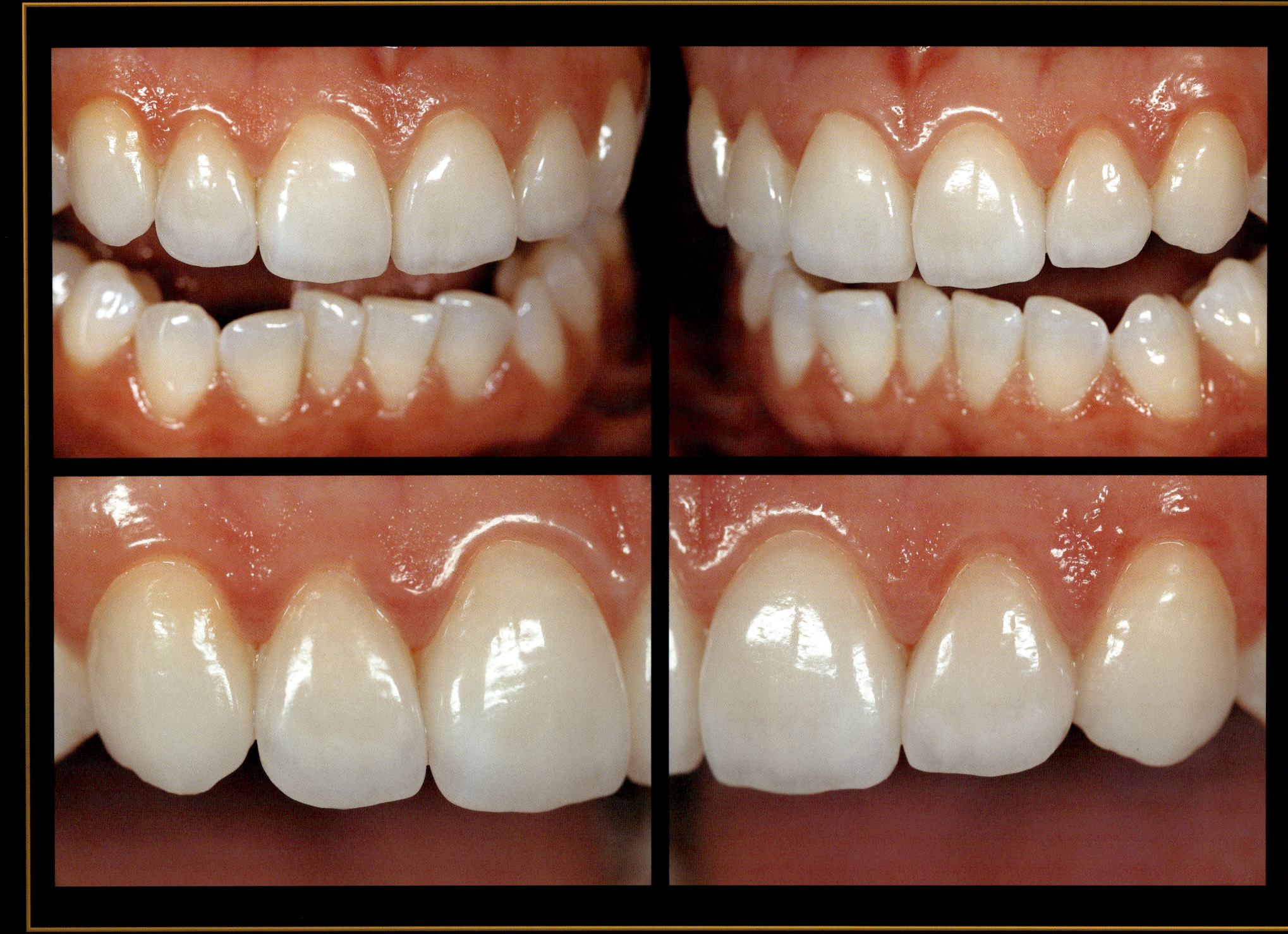

CASE 30

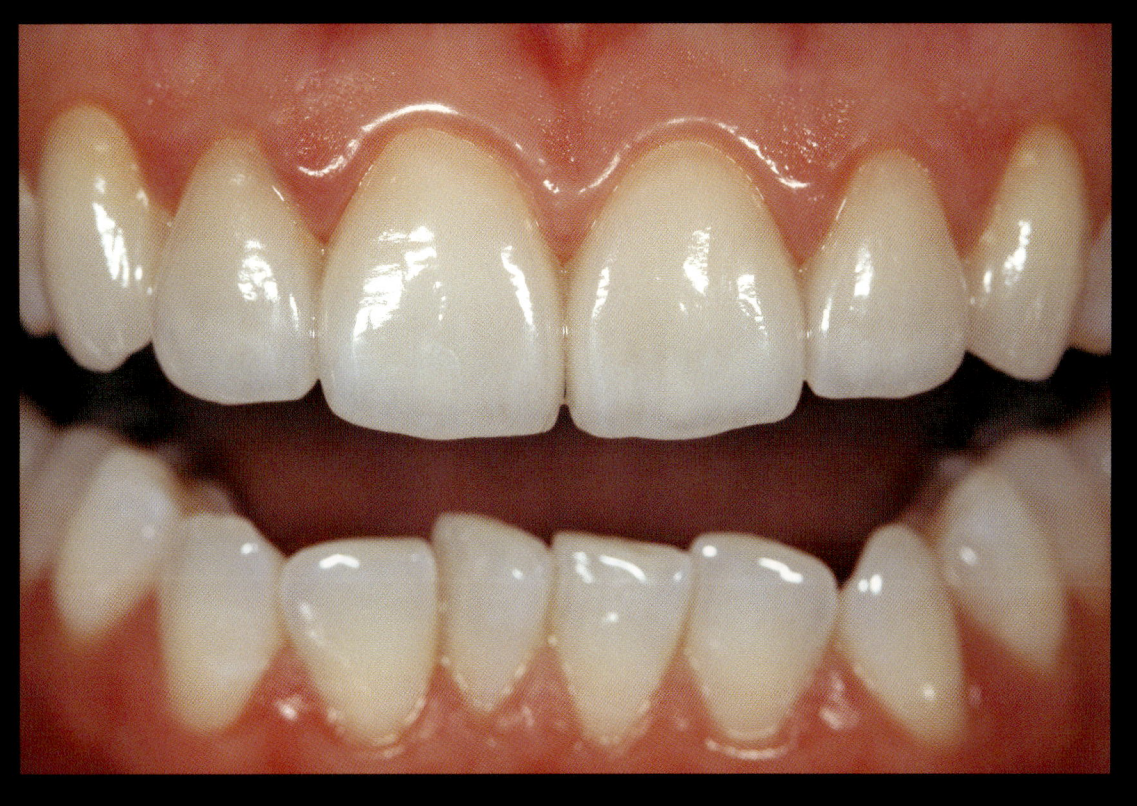

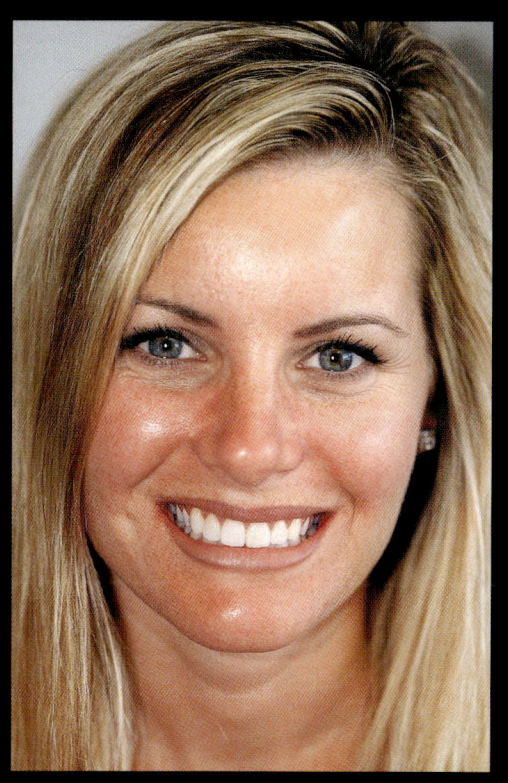

CASE 31

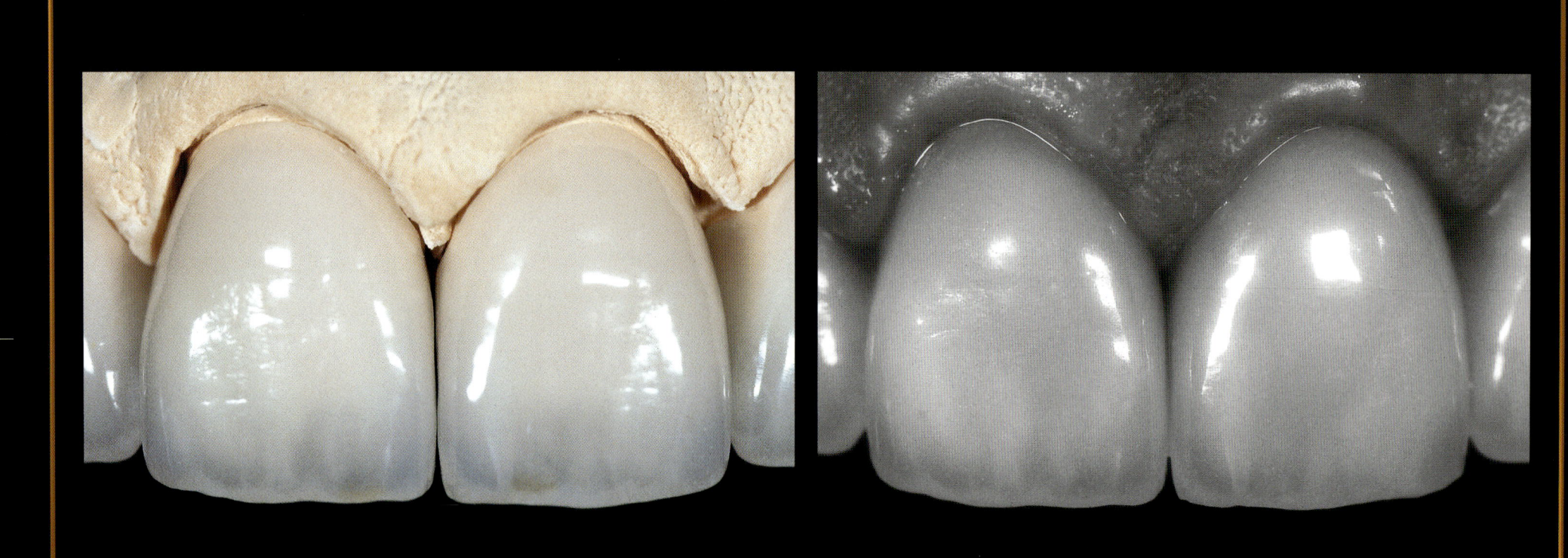

CASE 31

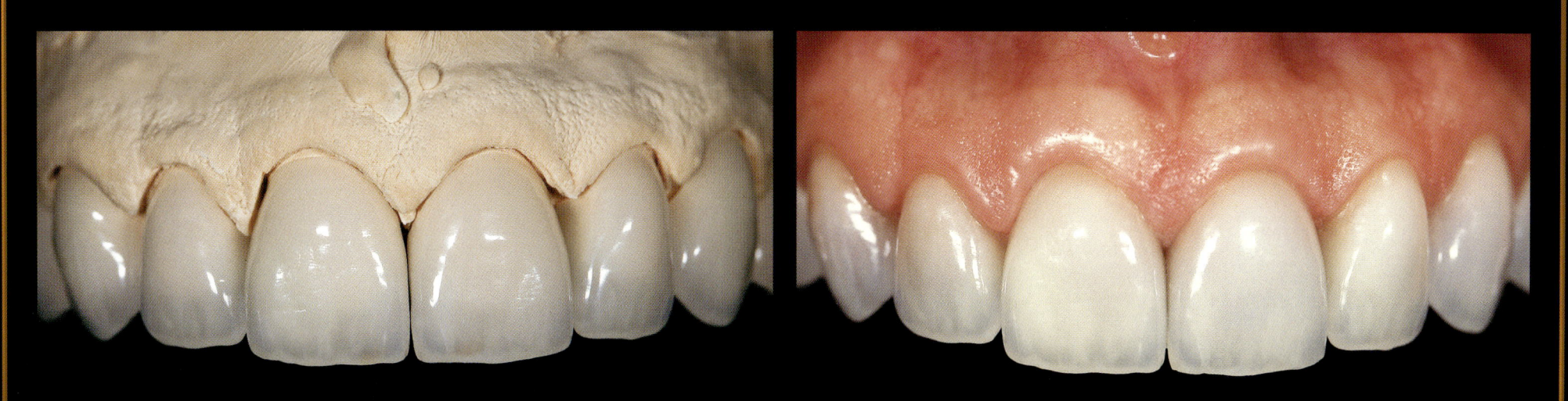

CASE 32

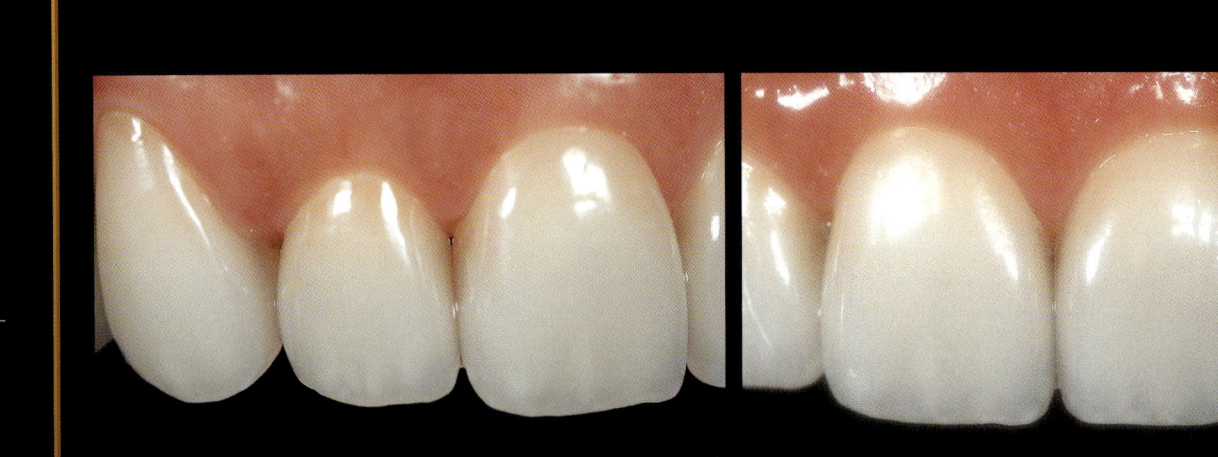

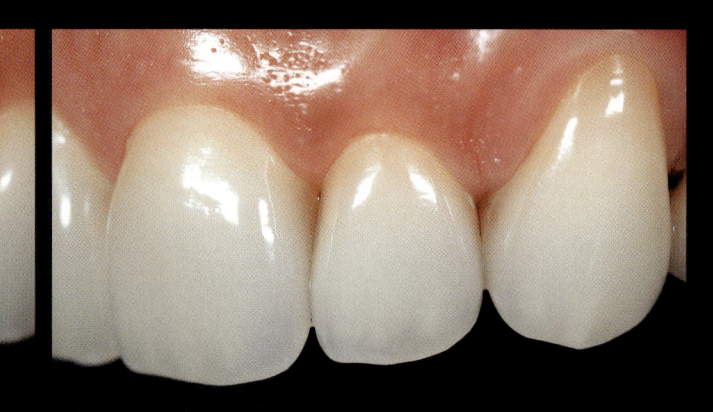

83

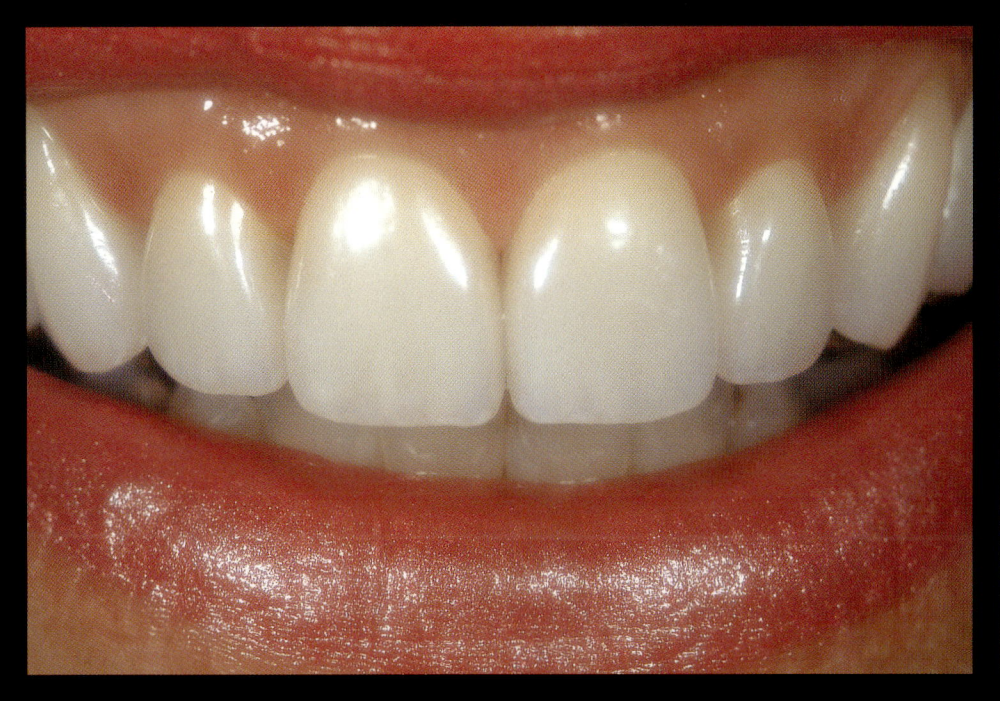

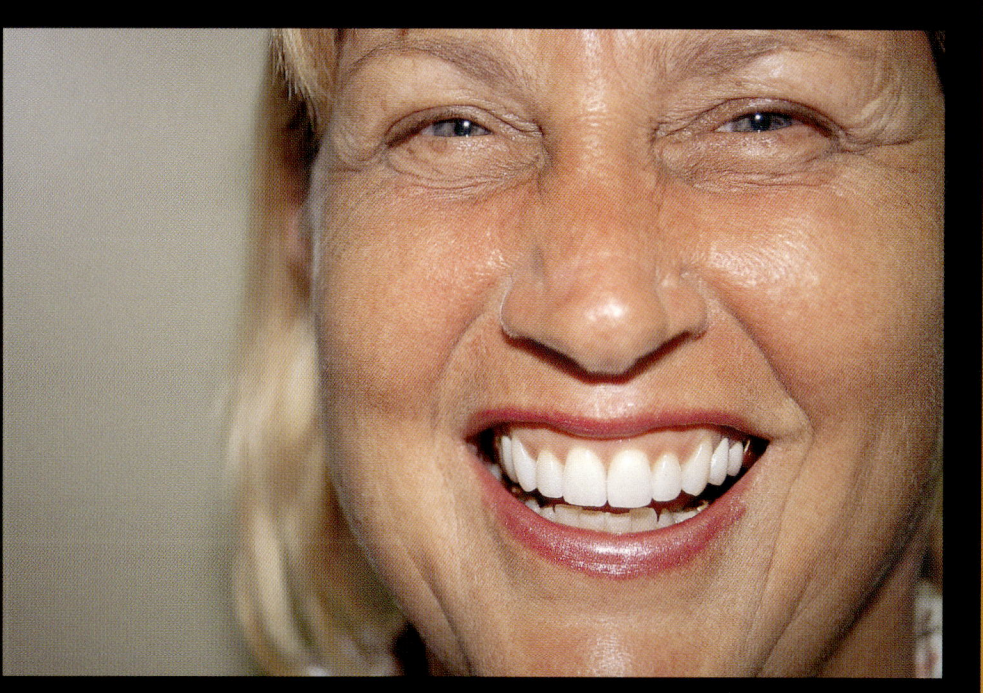

CASE 33

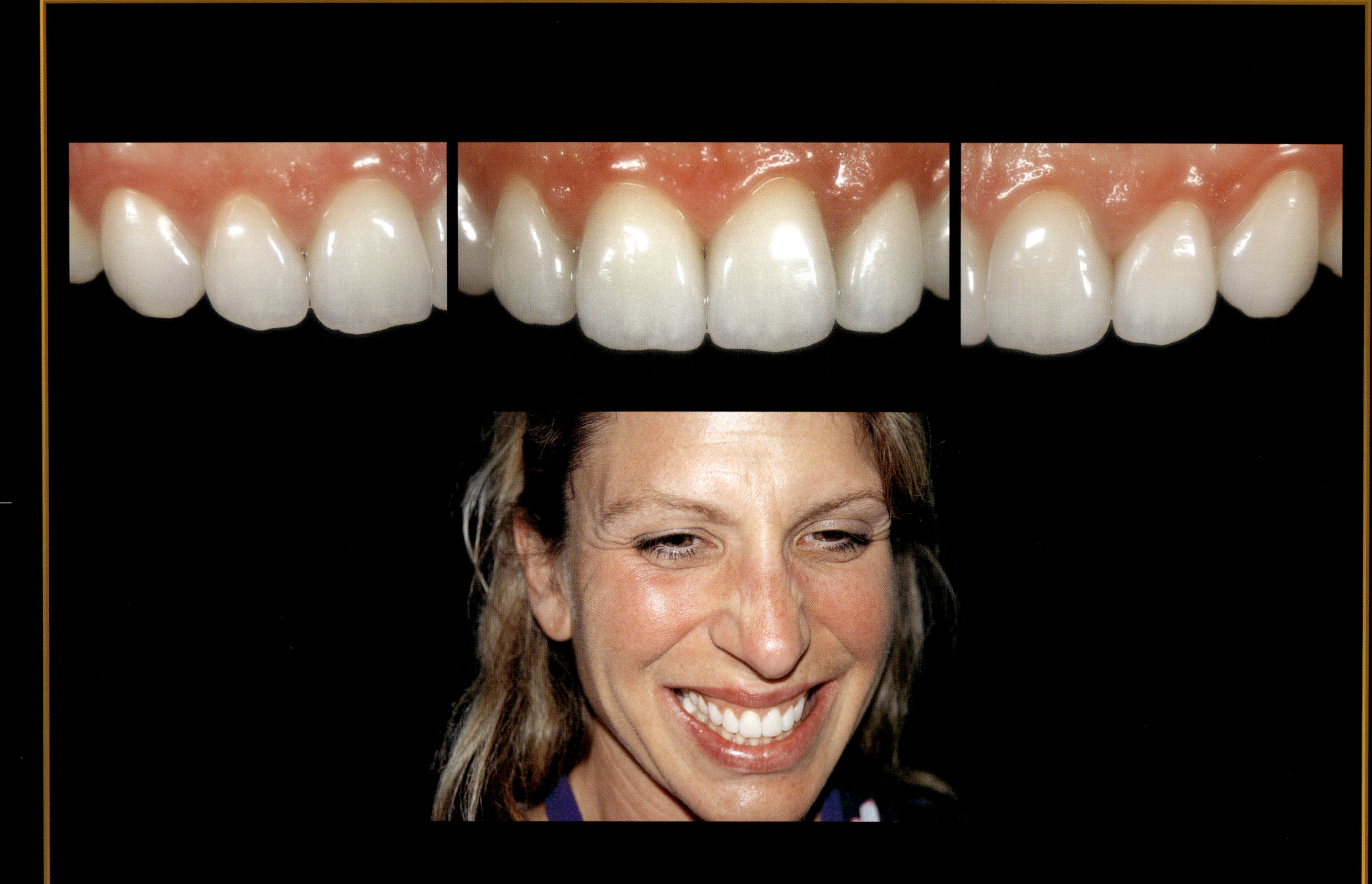

CASE 34

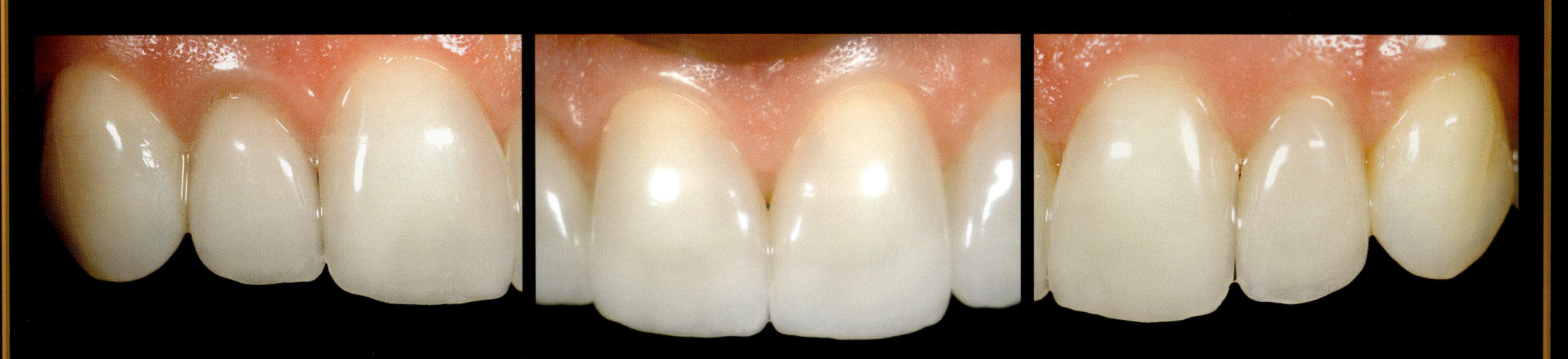

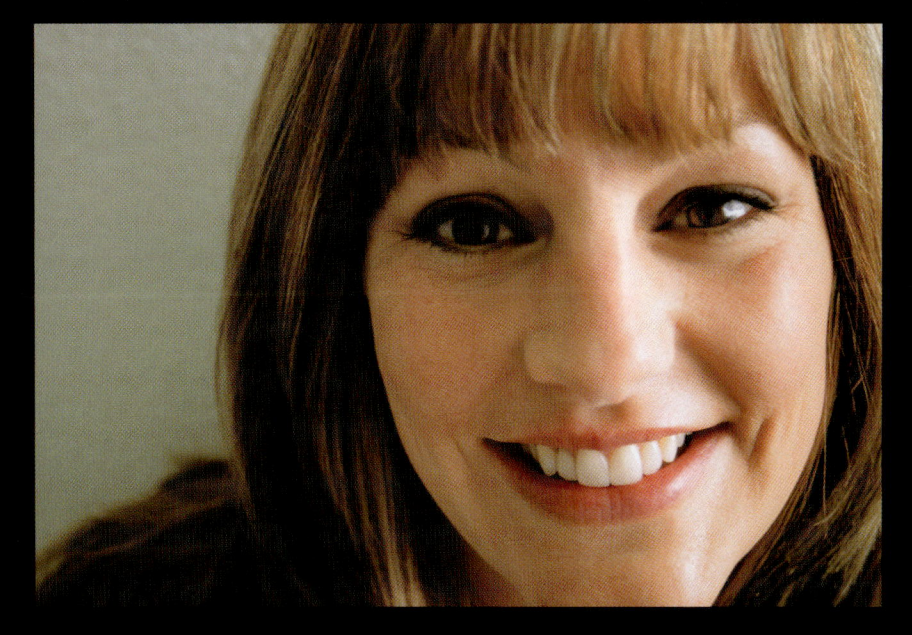

CASE 35

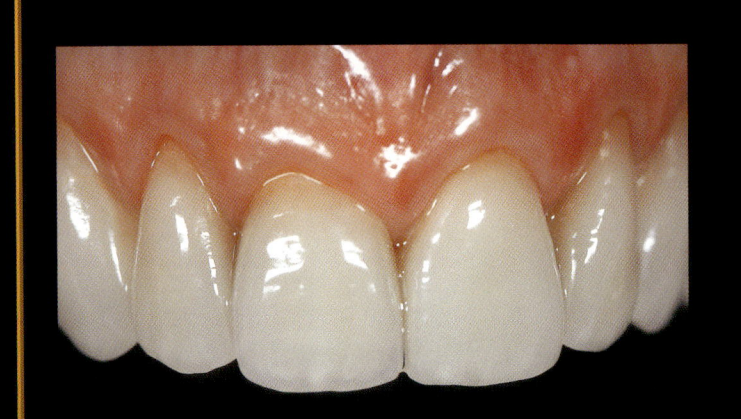

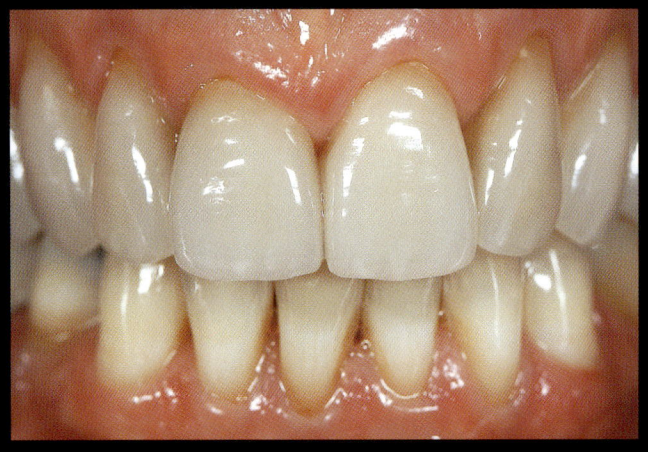

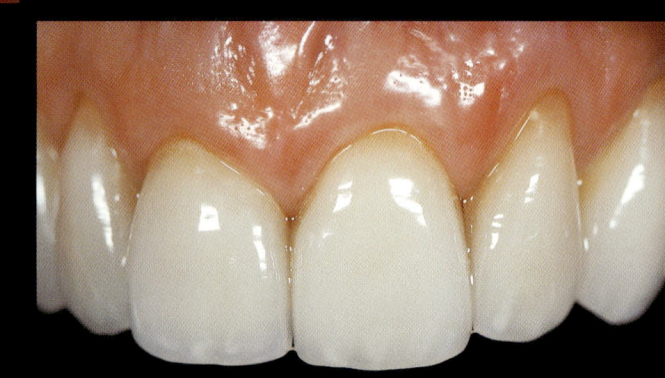

CASE 36

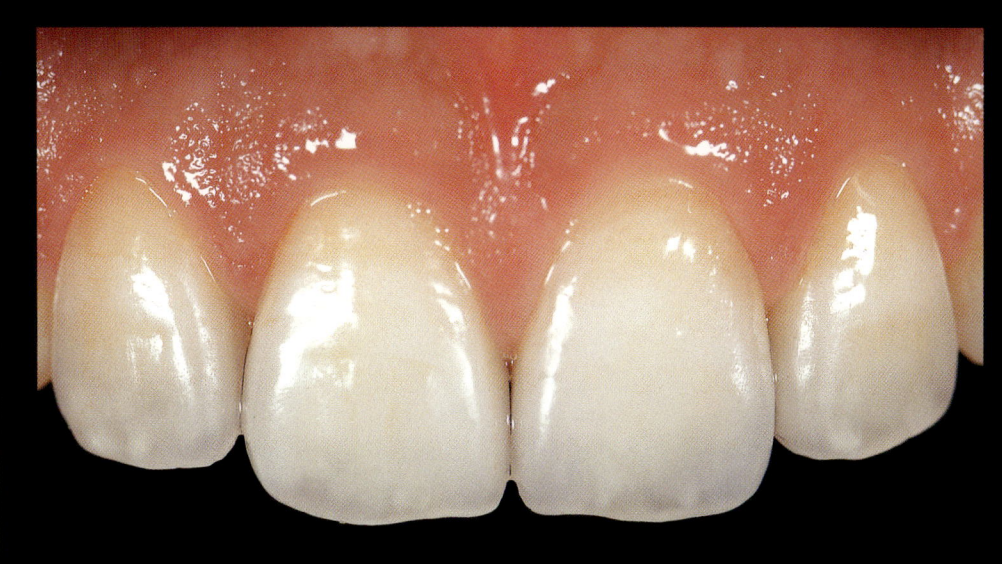

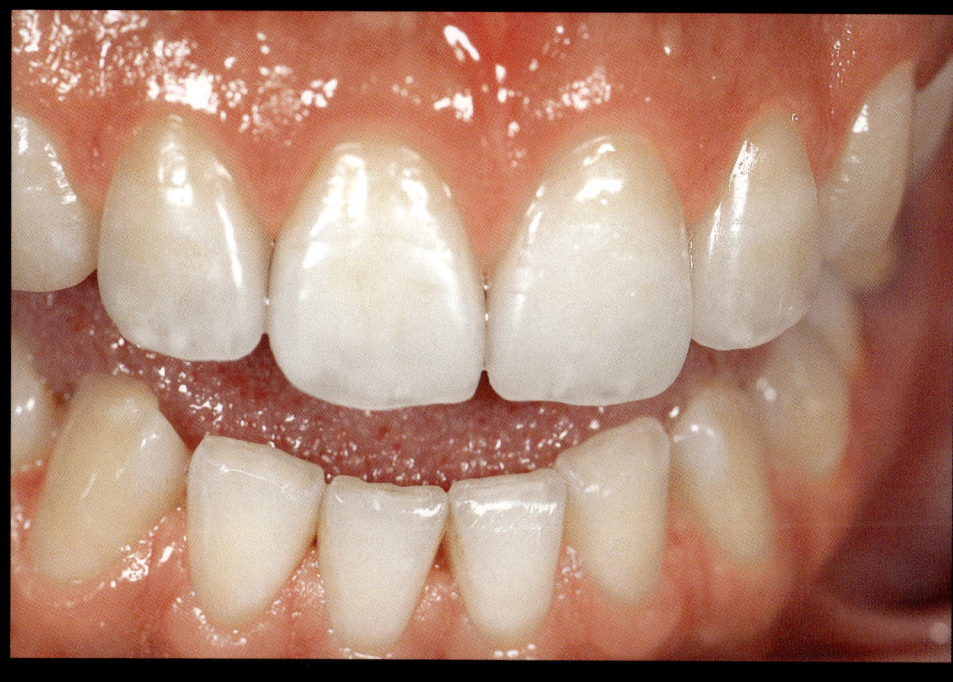

CASE 37

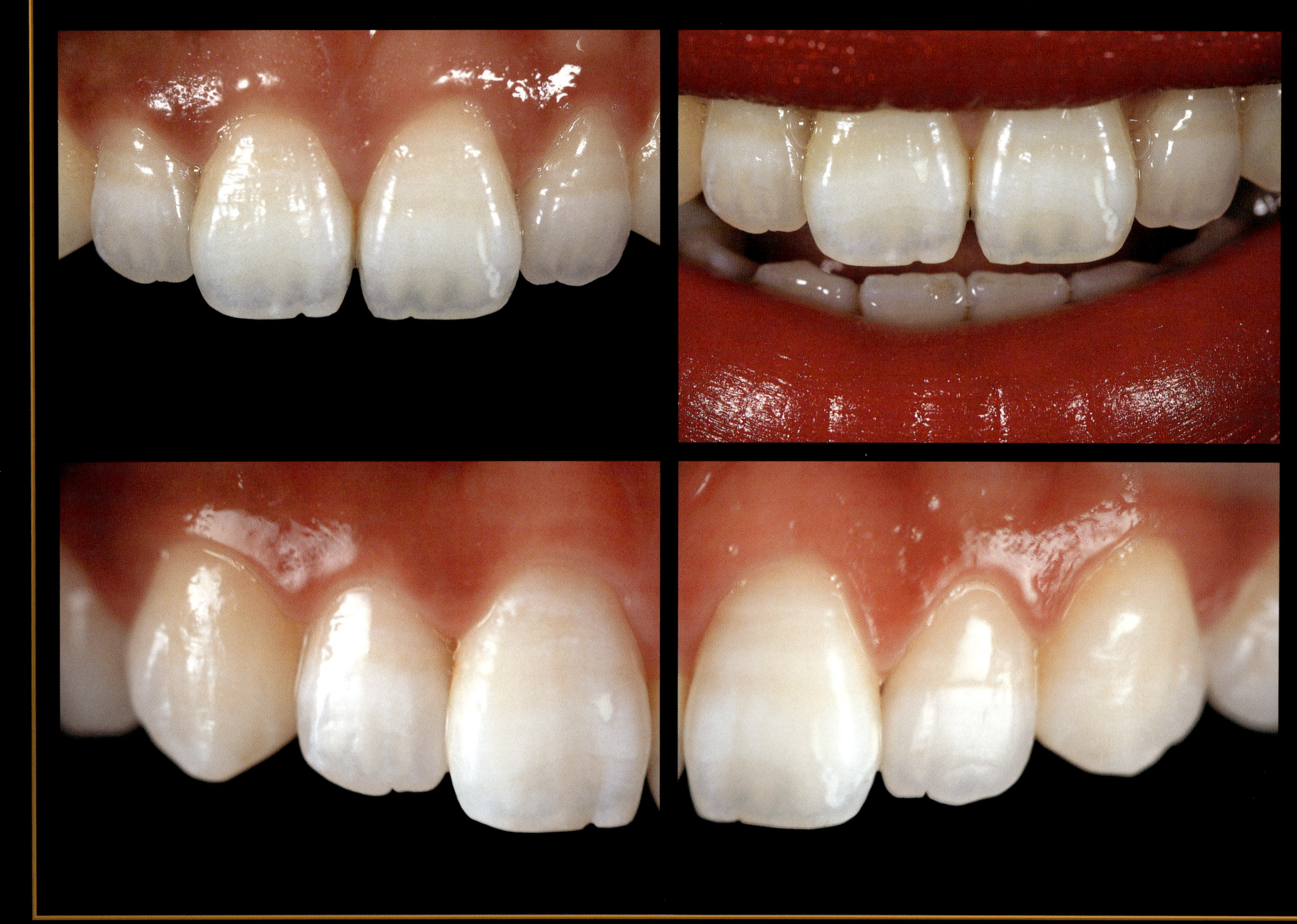

CASE 37

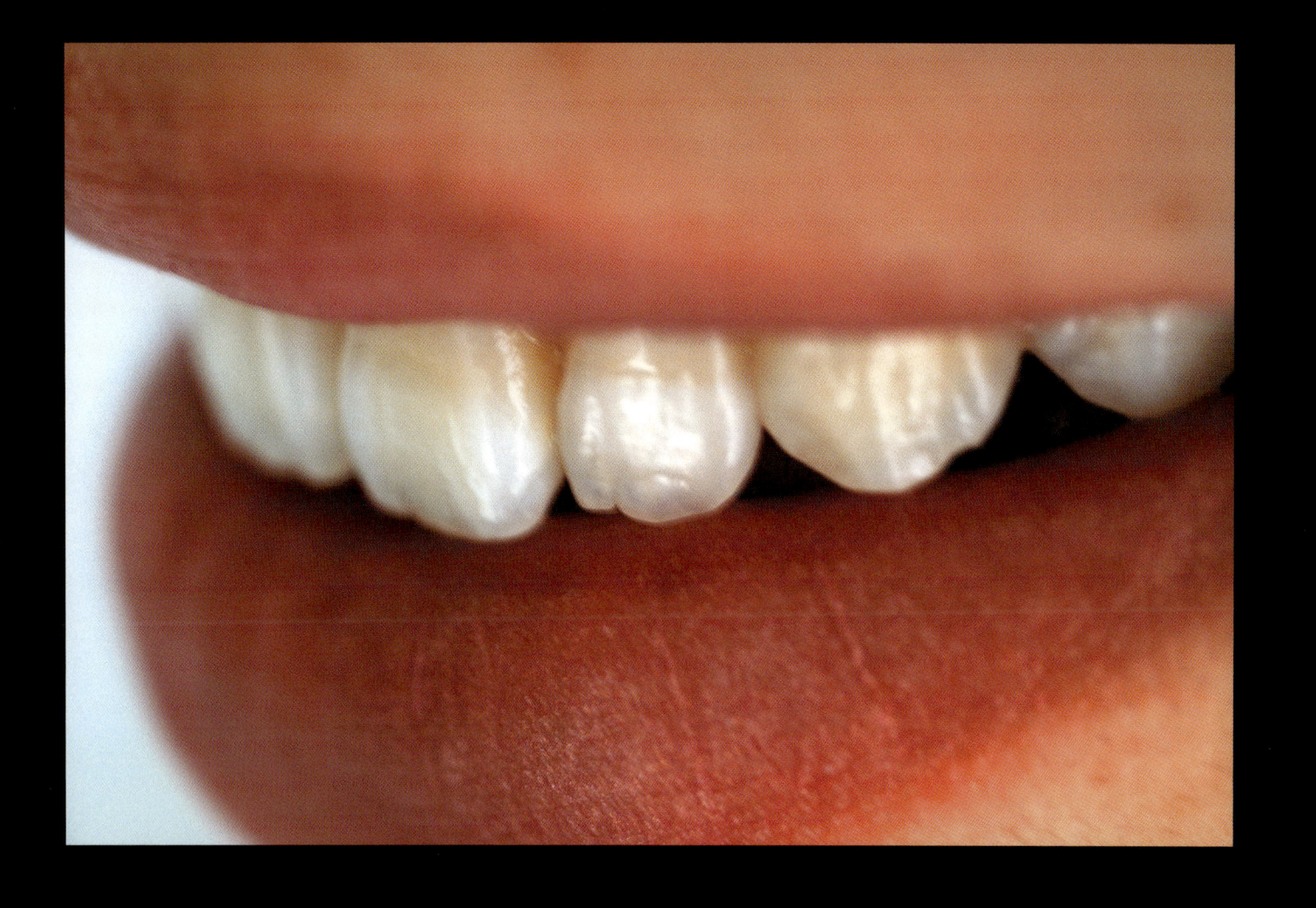

CASE 38

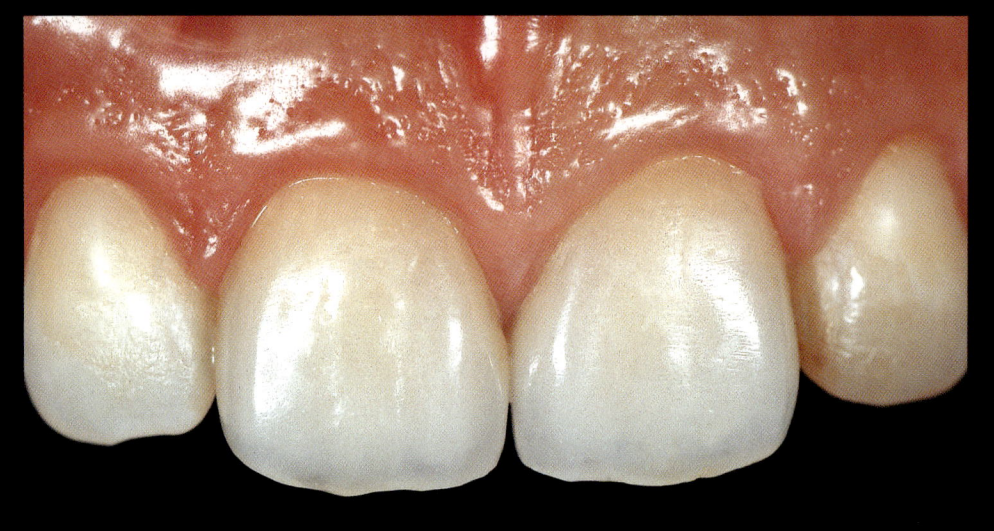

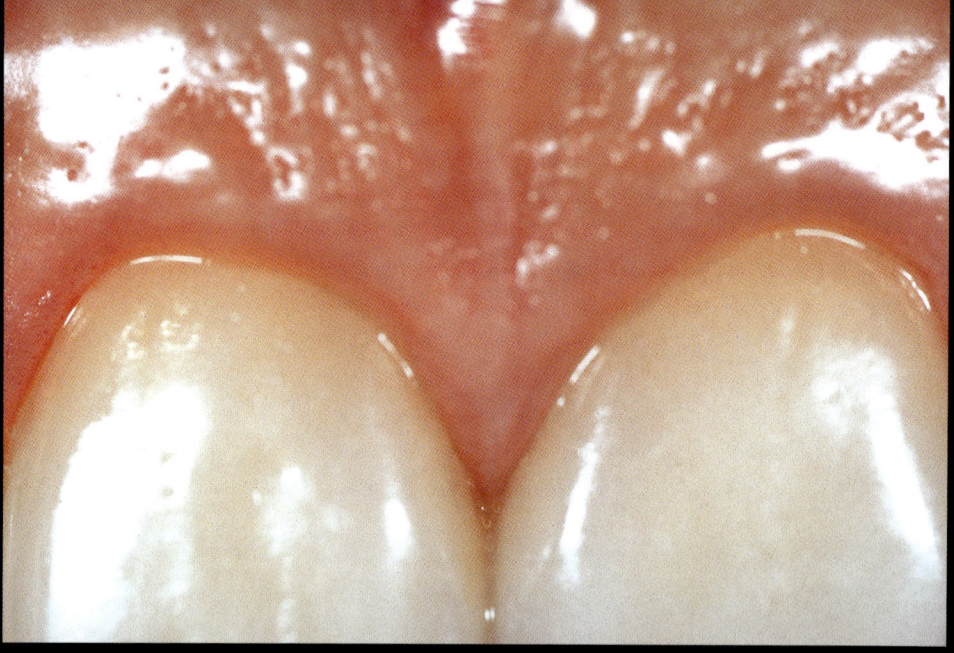

CASE 39

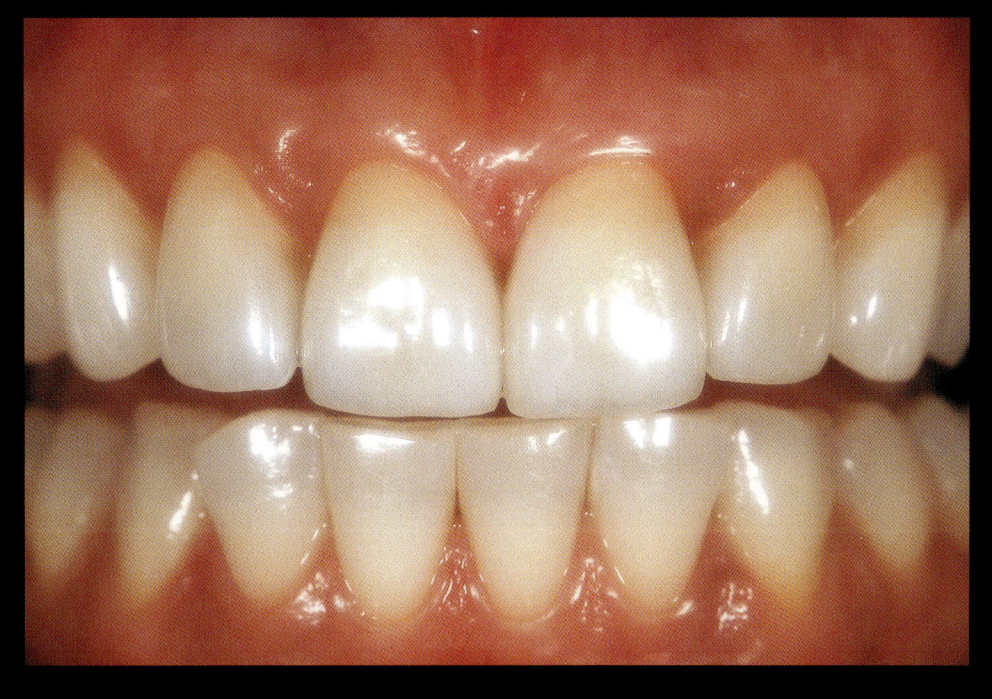

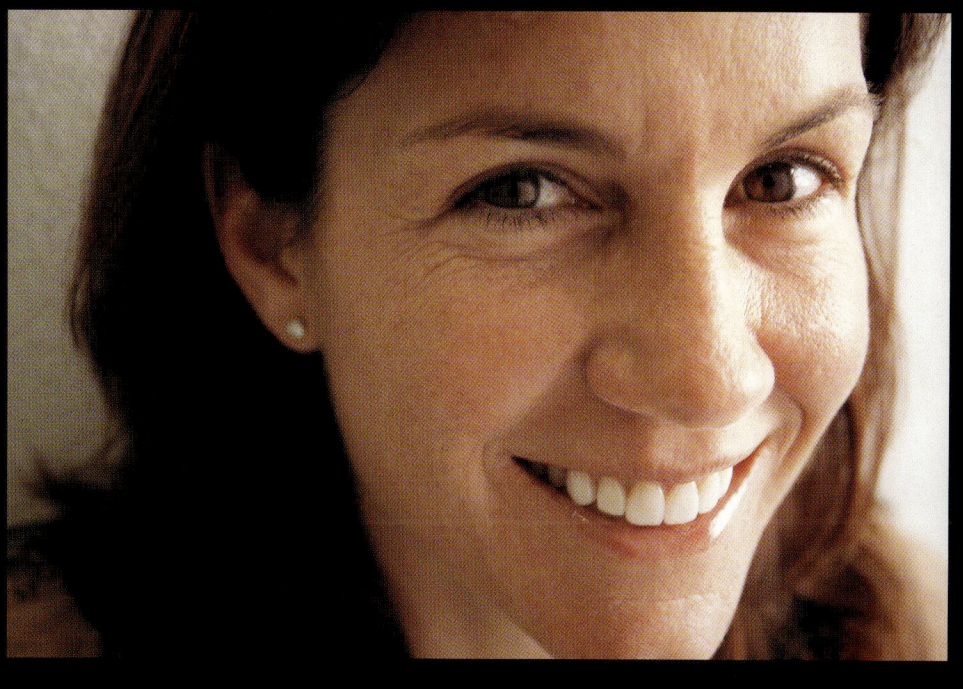

CASE 40

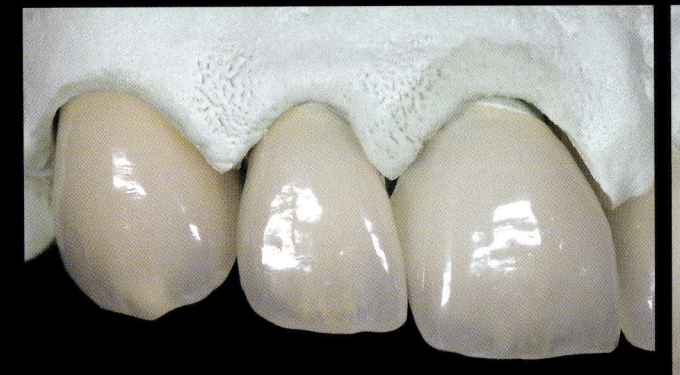

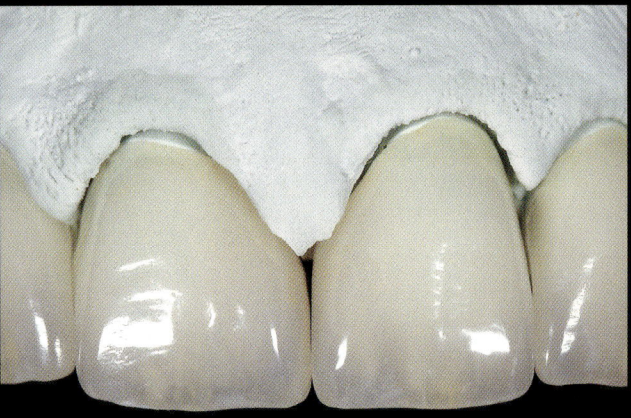

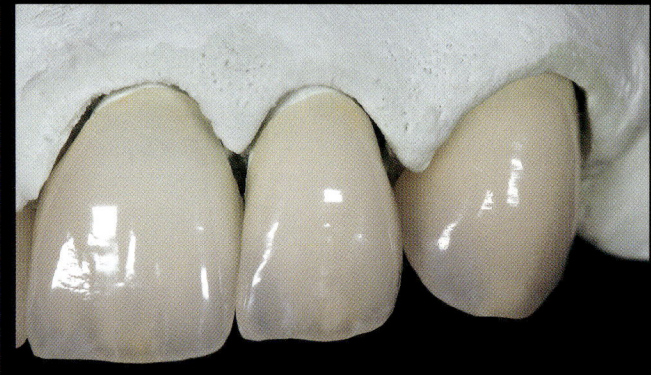

CASE 40

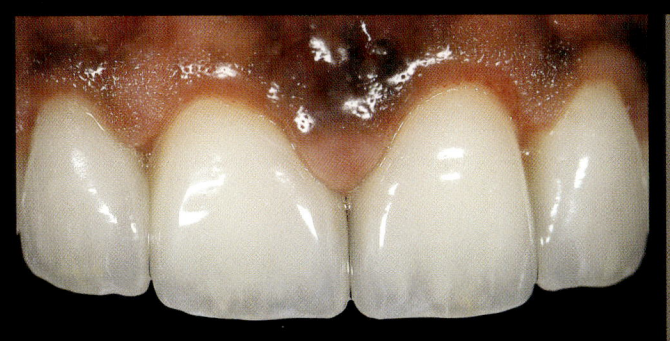

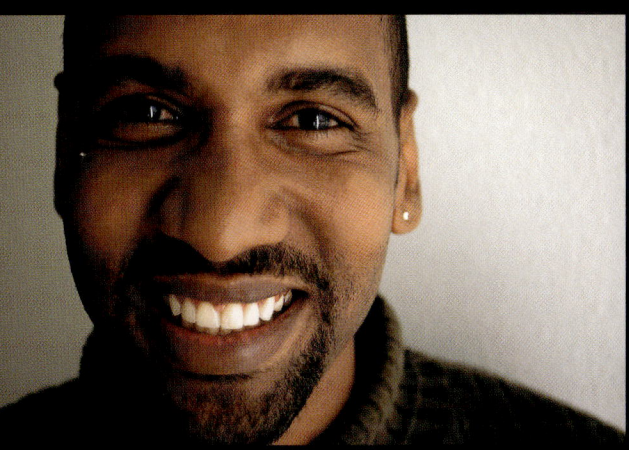

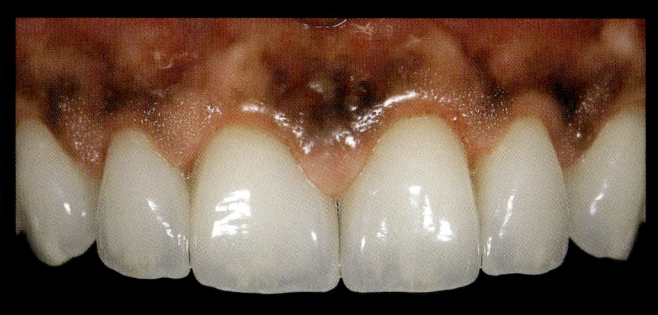

CASE 41

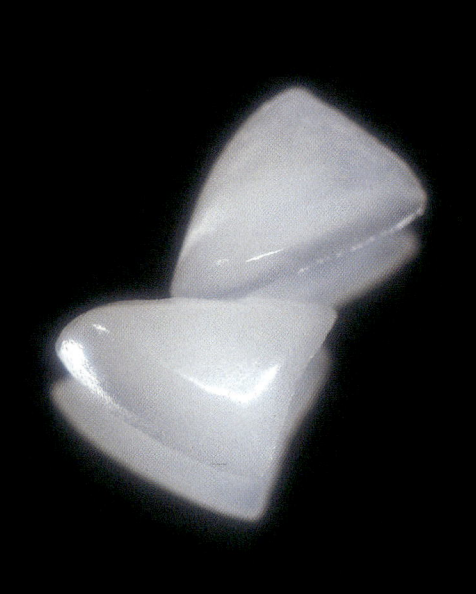

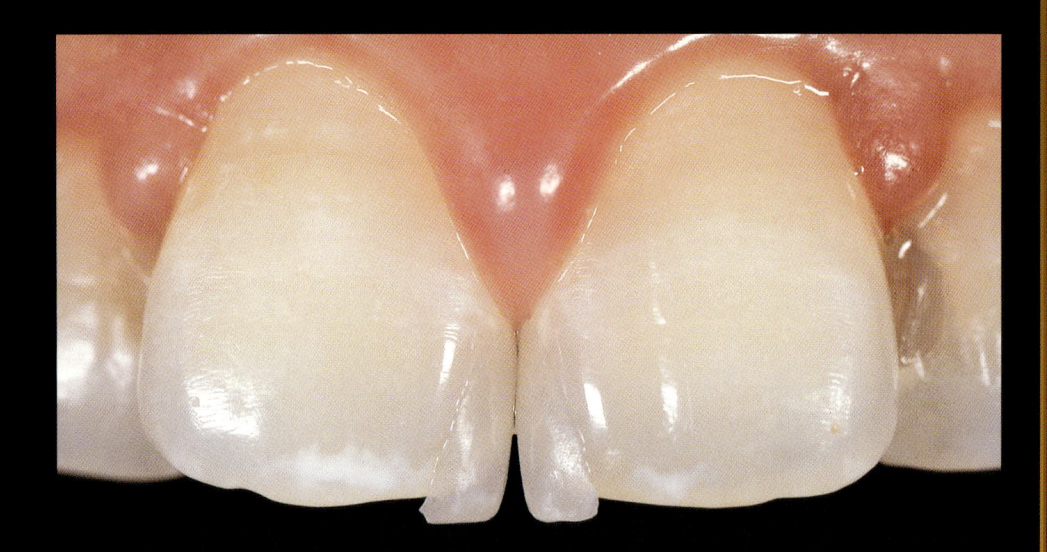

CASE 41

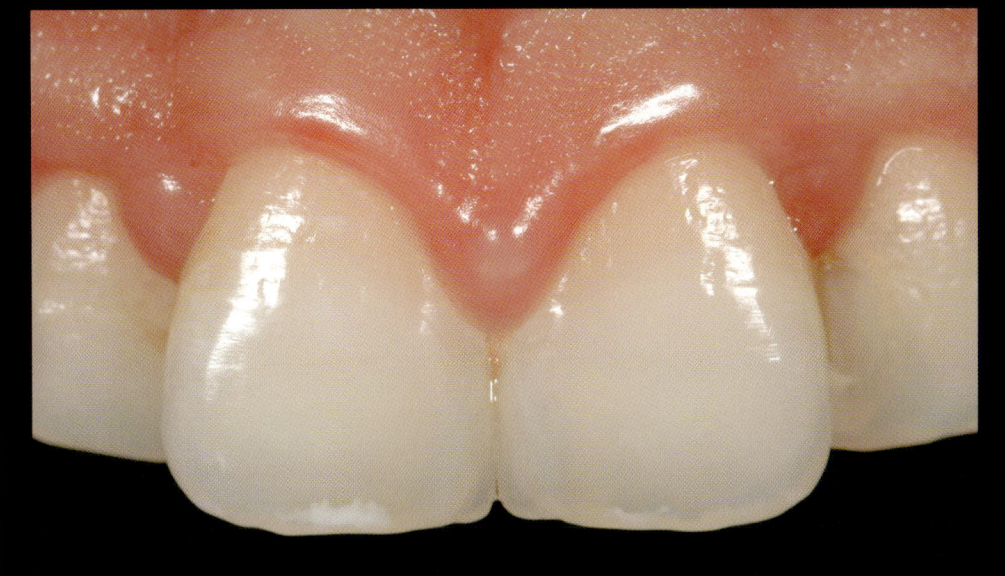

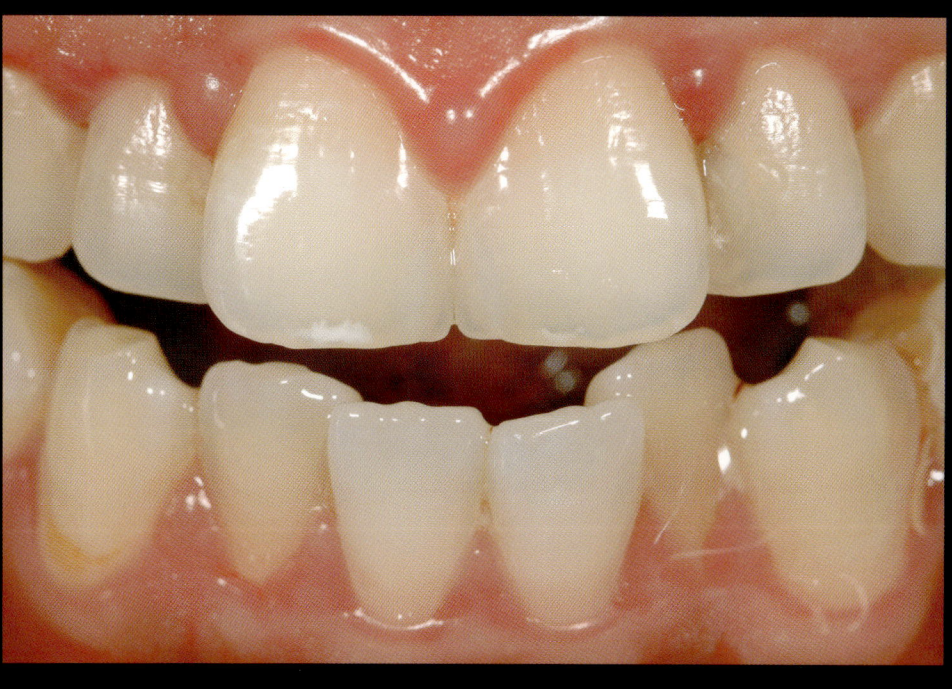

CASE 42

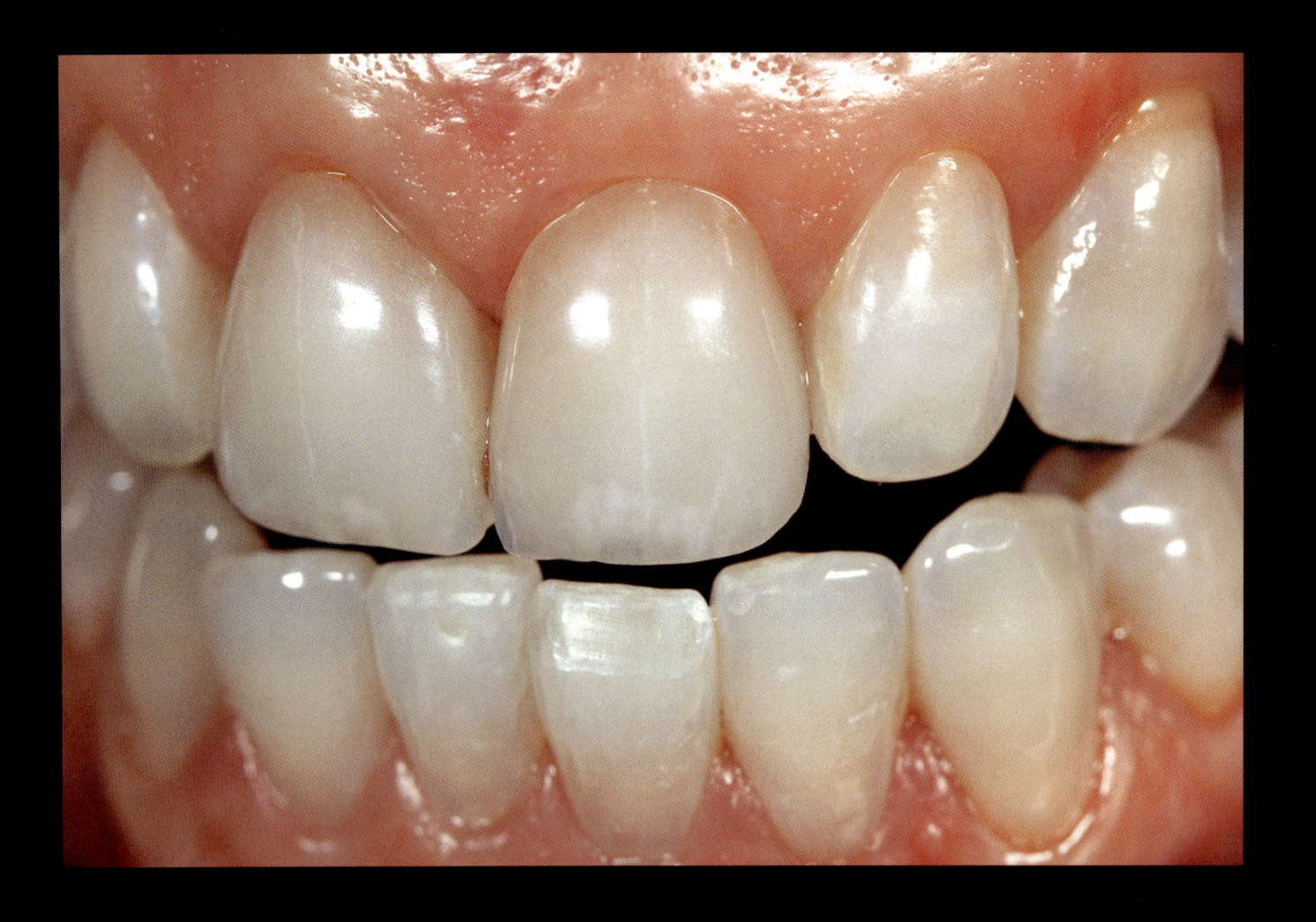

CASE 42

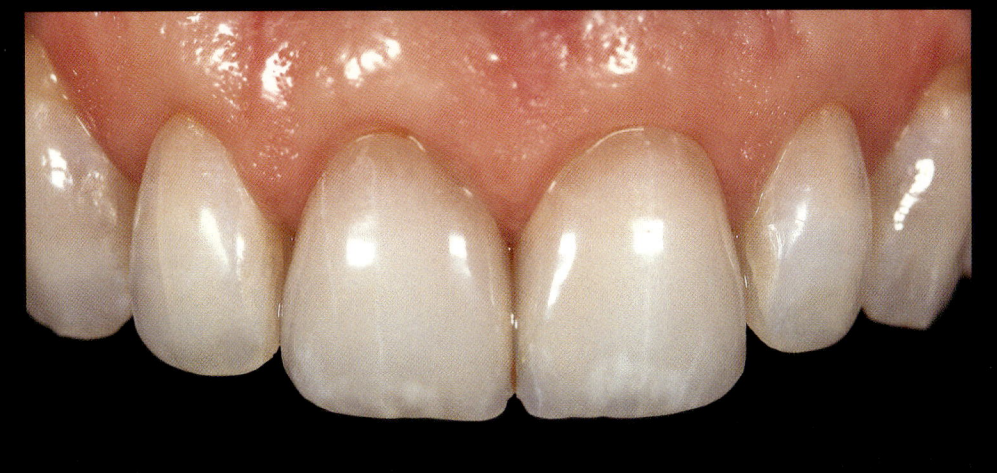

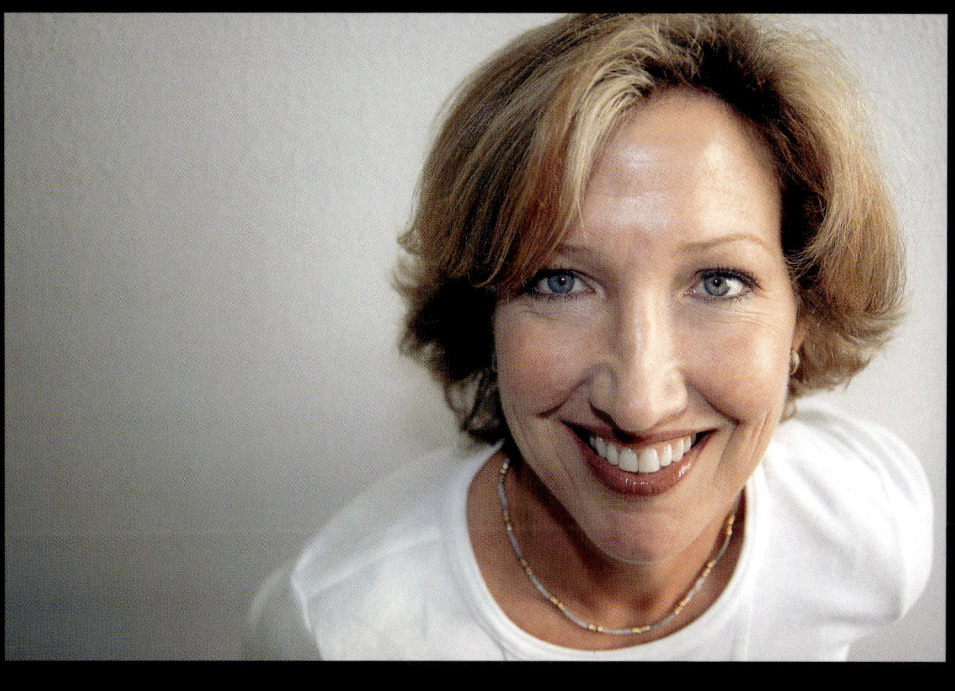

CASE 43

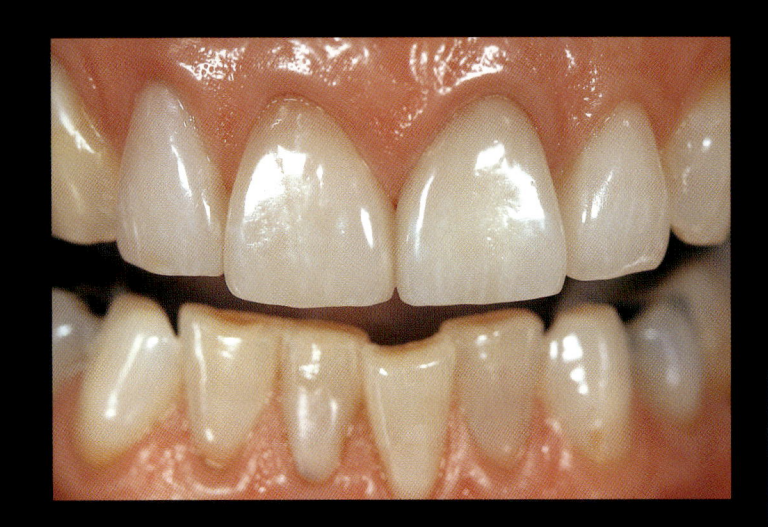

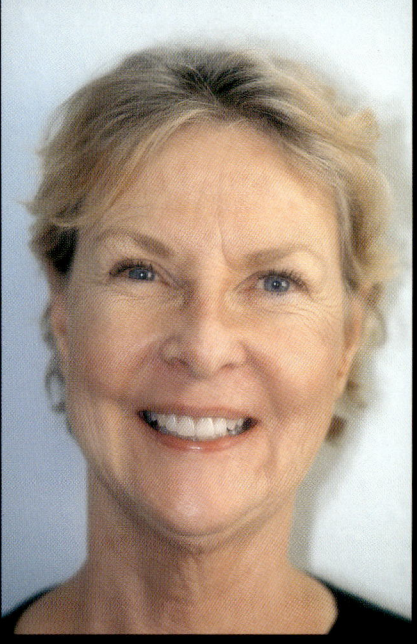

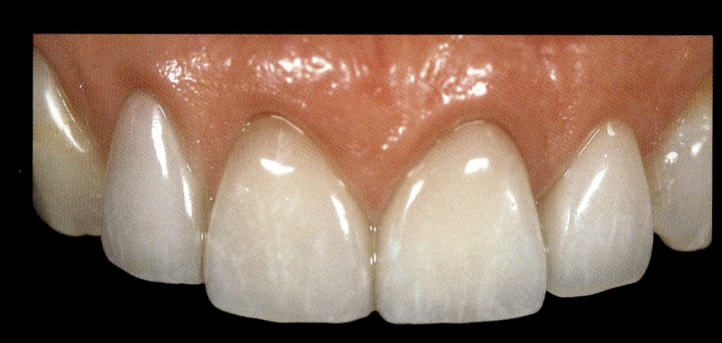

CASE 44

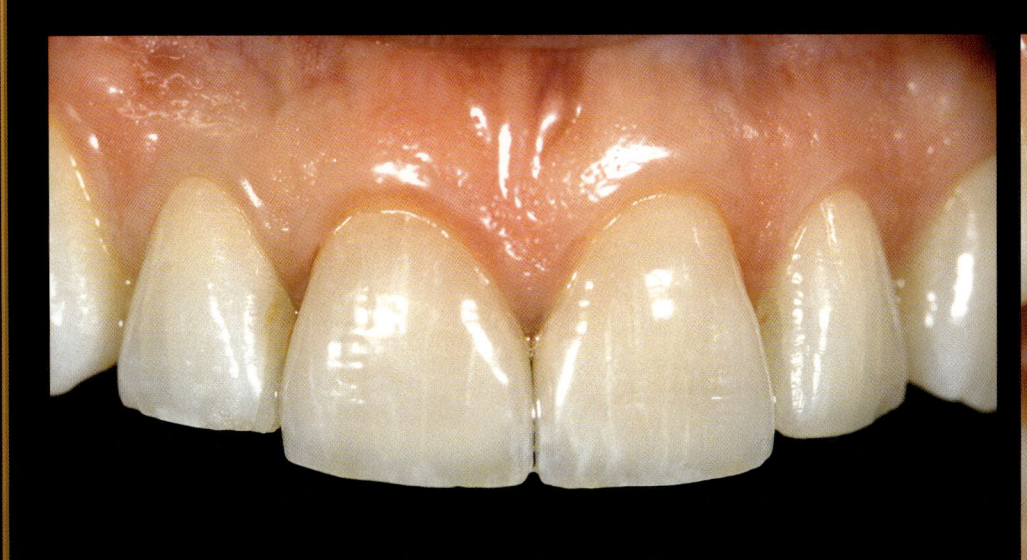

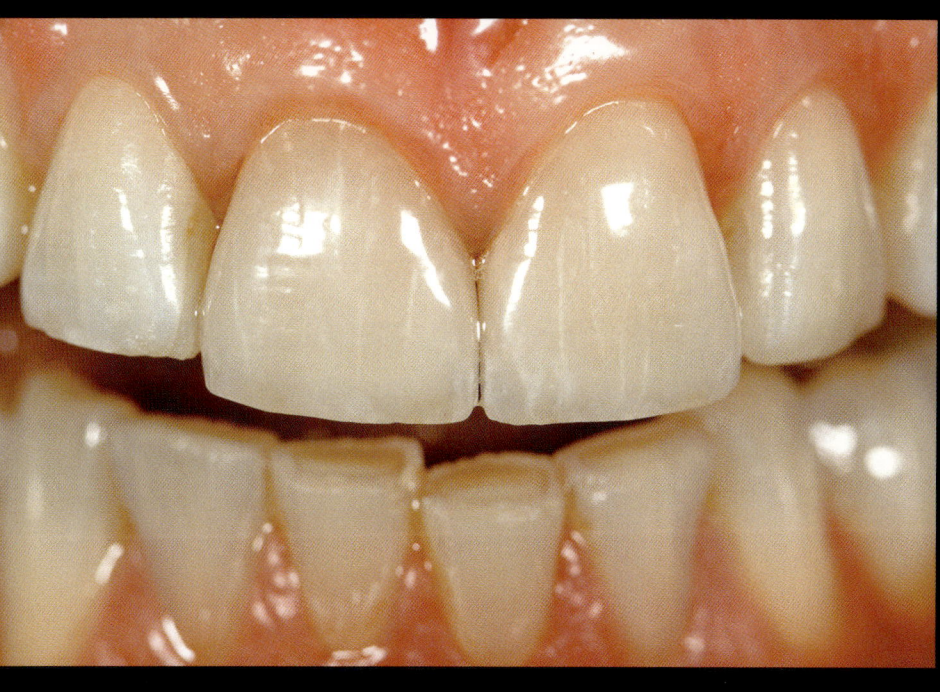

100

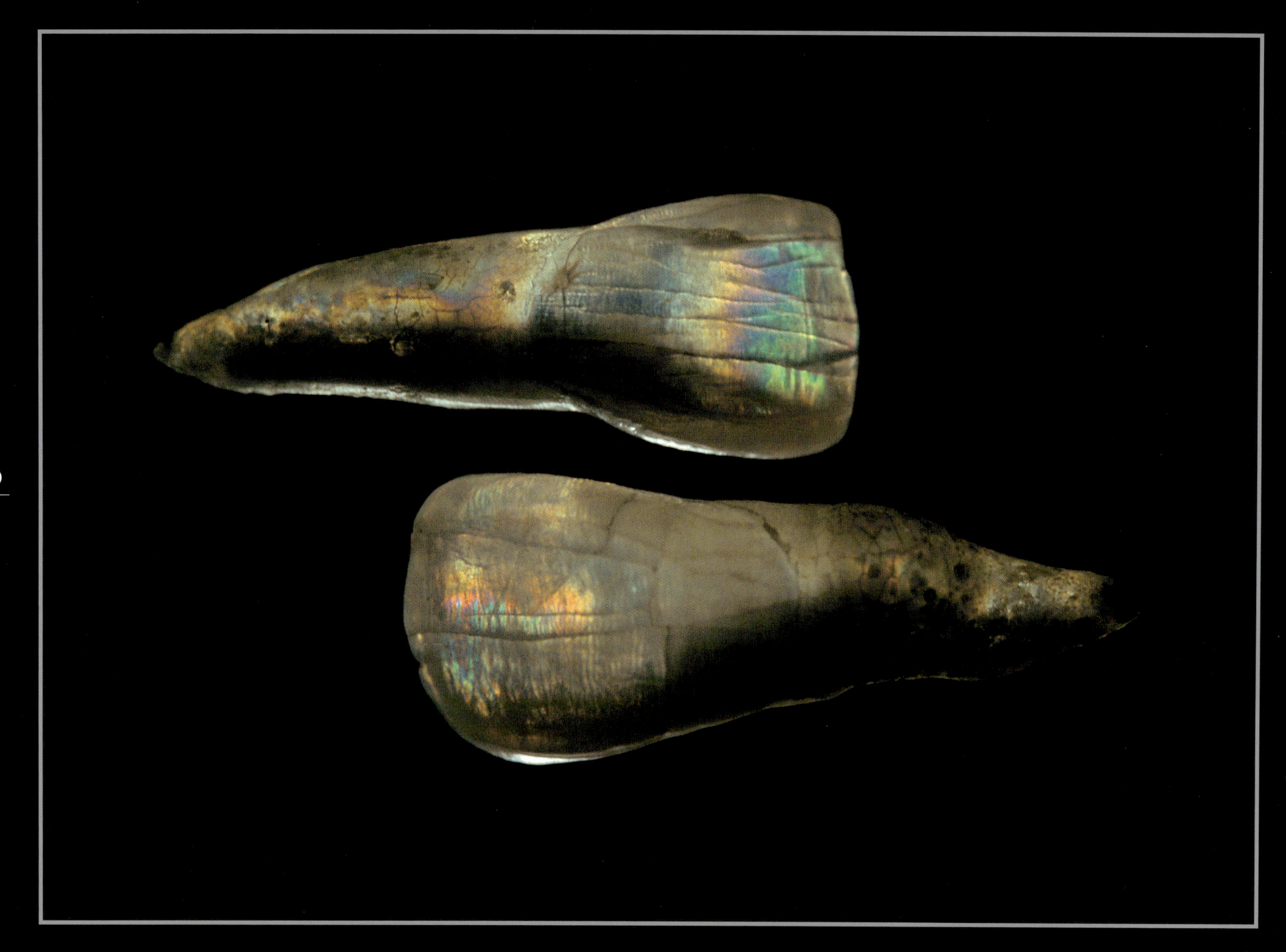

101

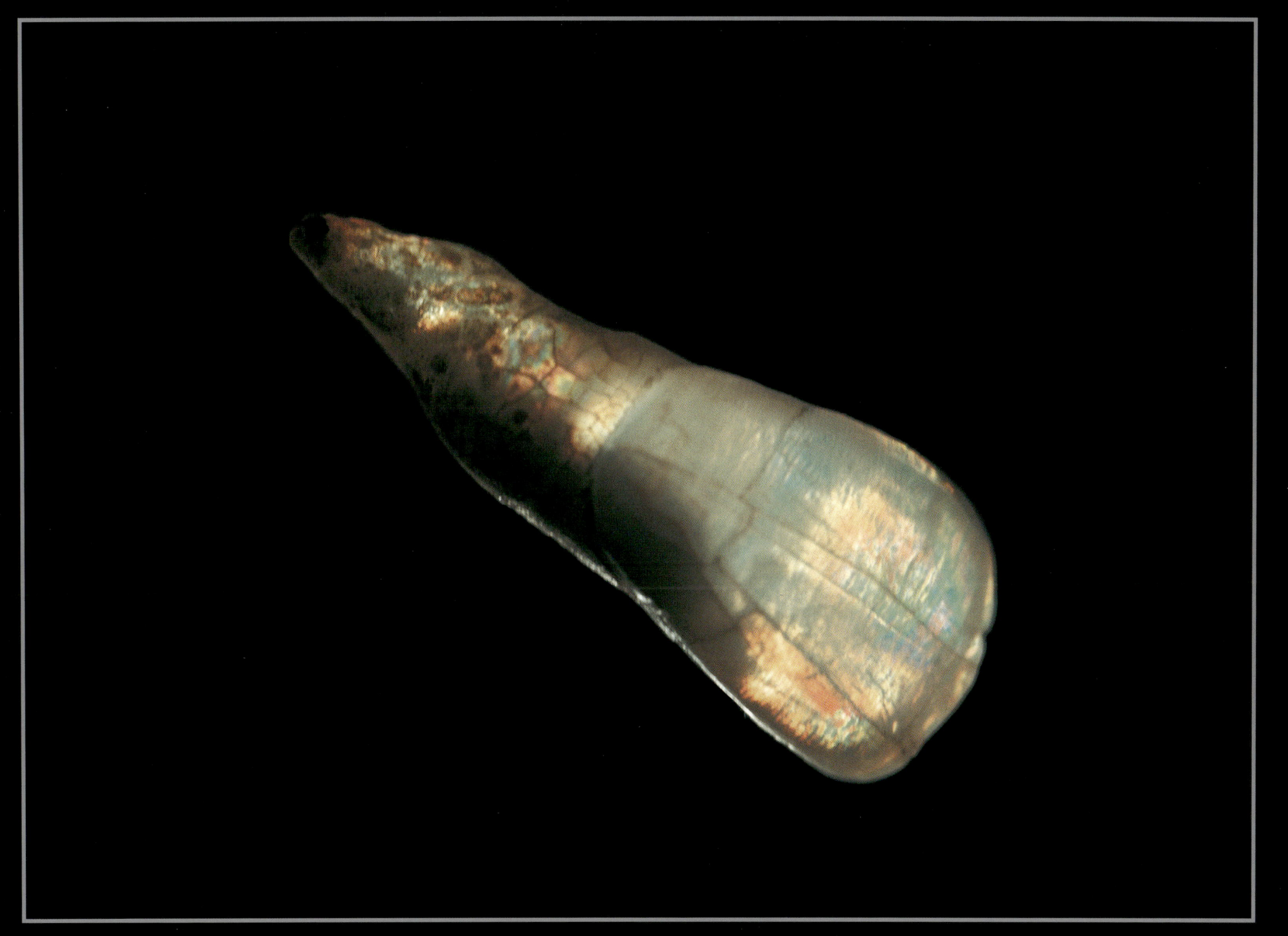

102

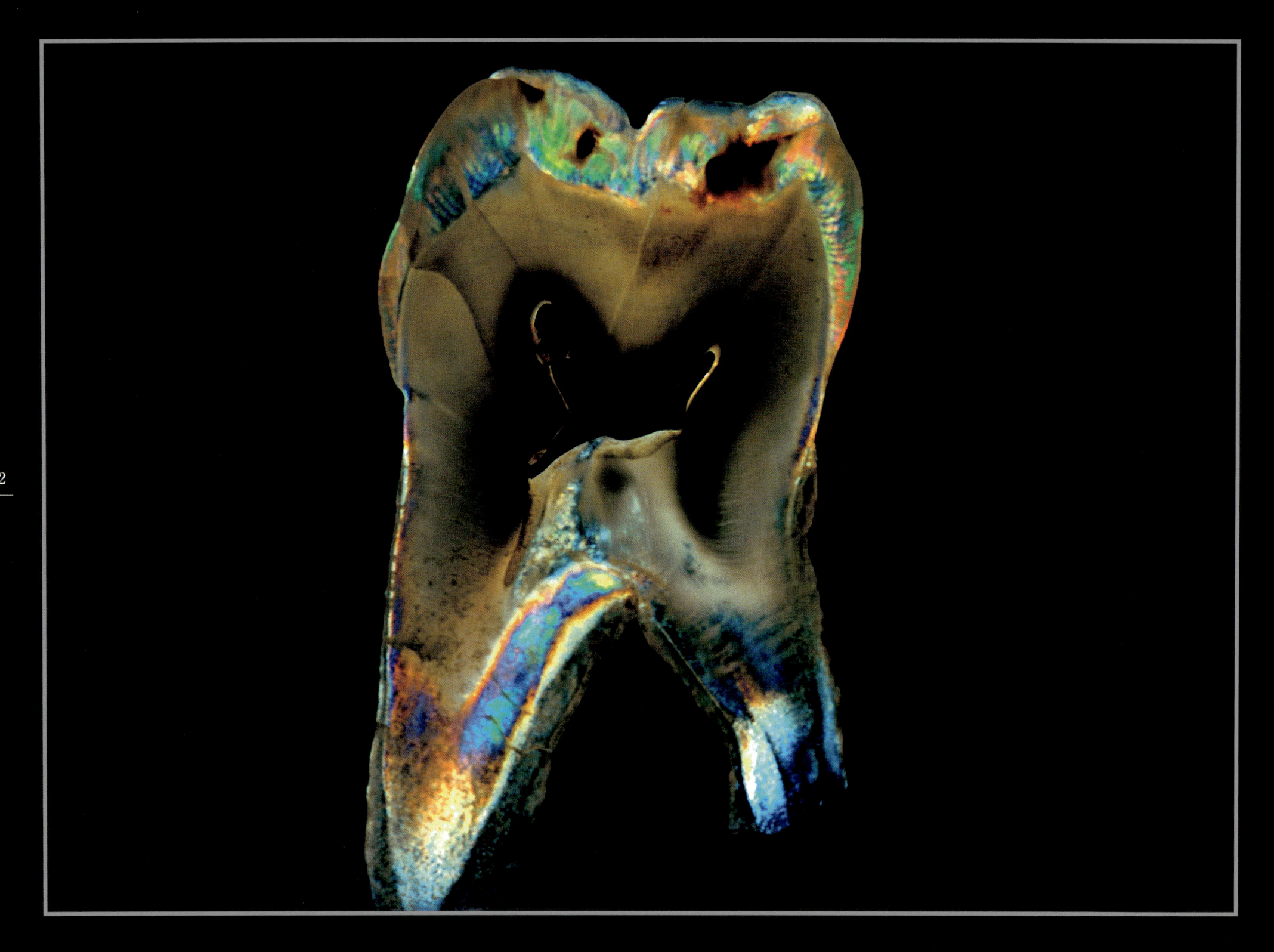

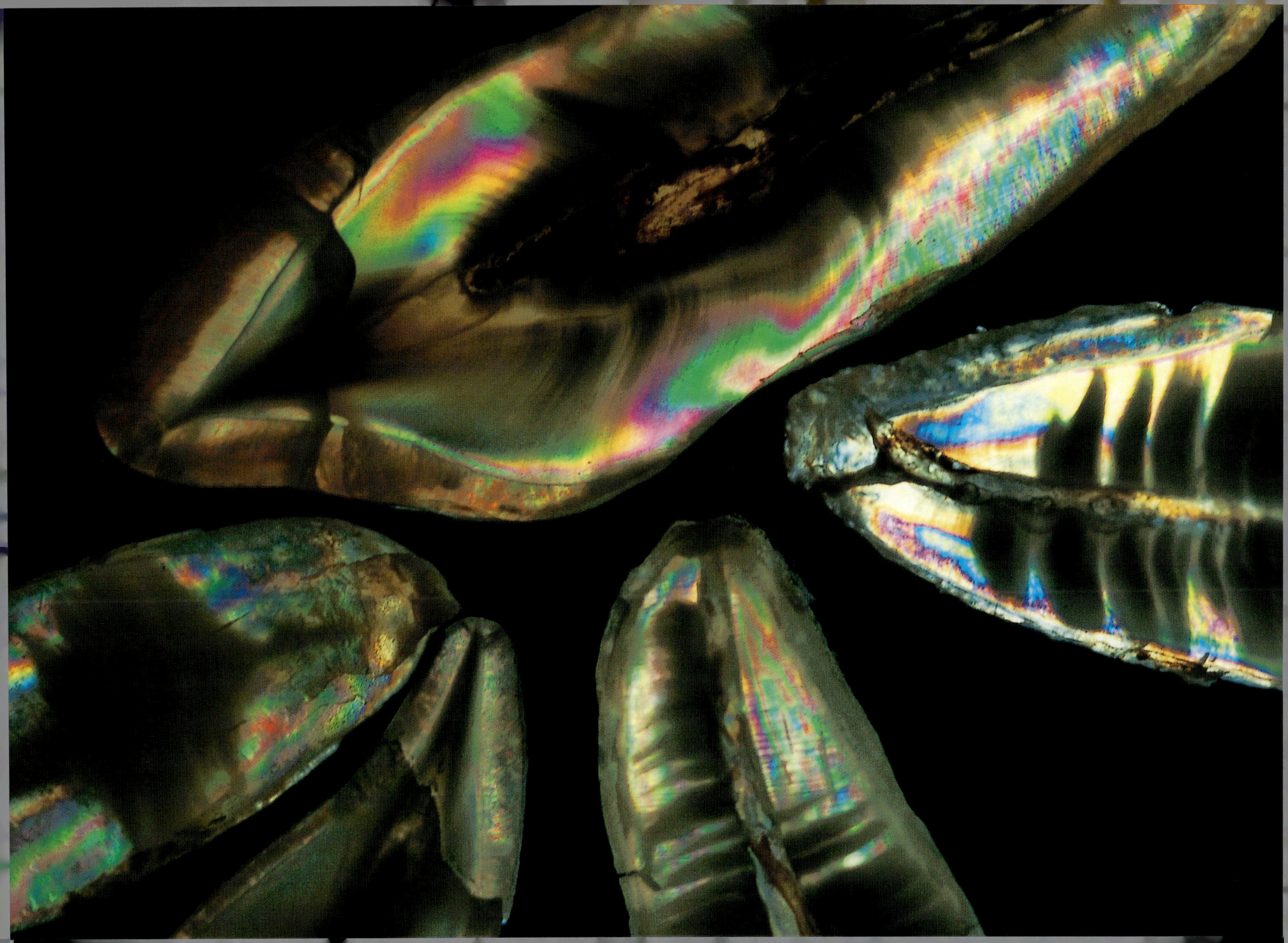

104

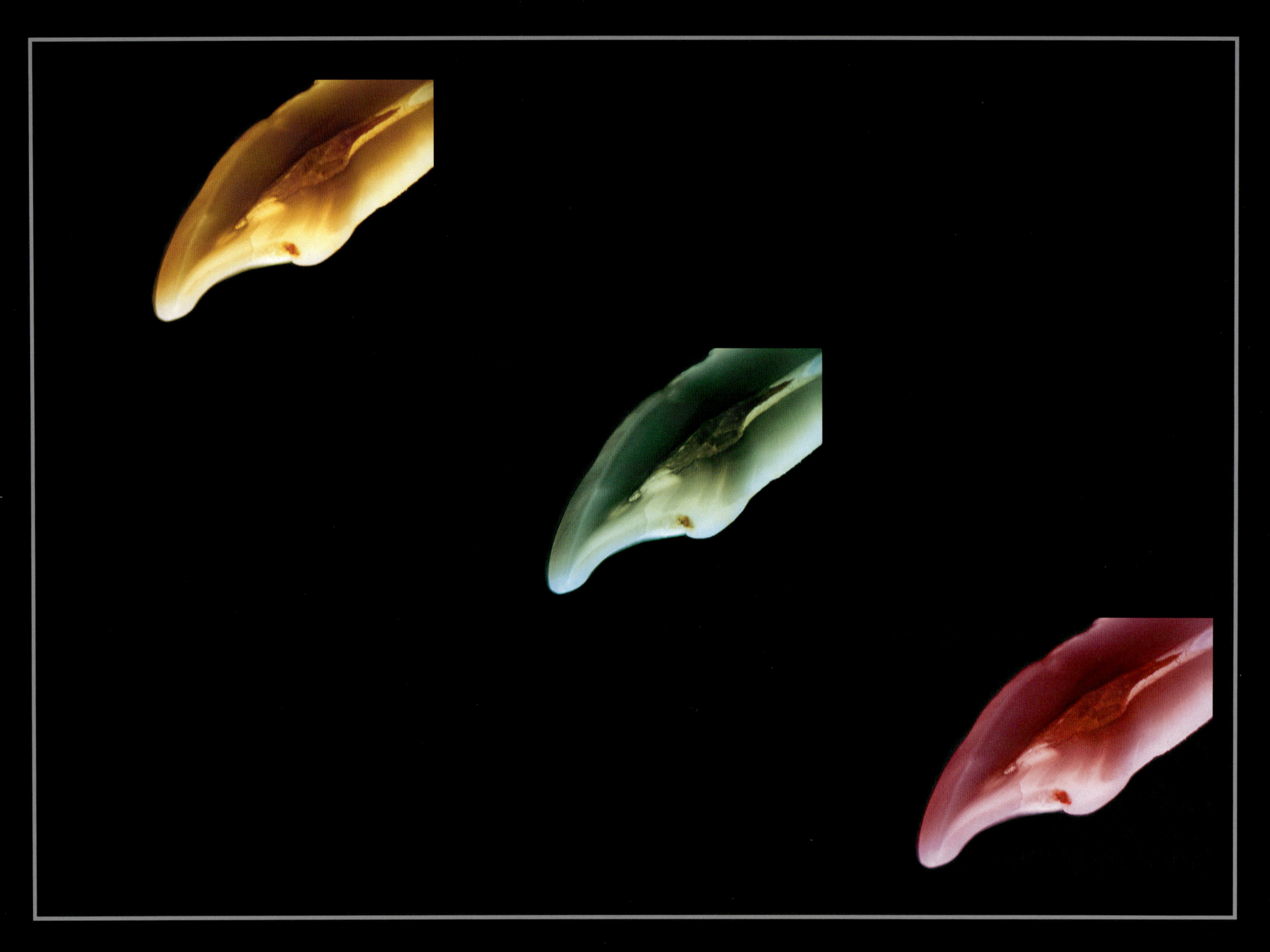

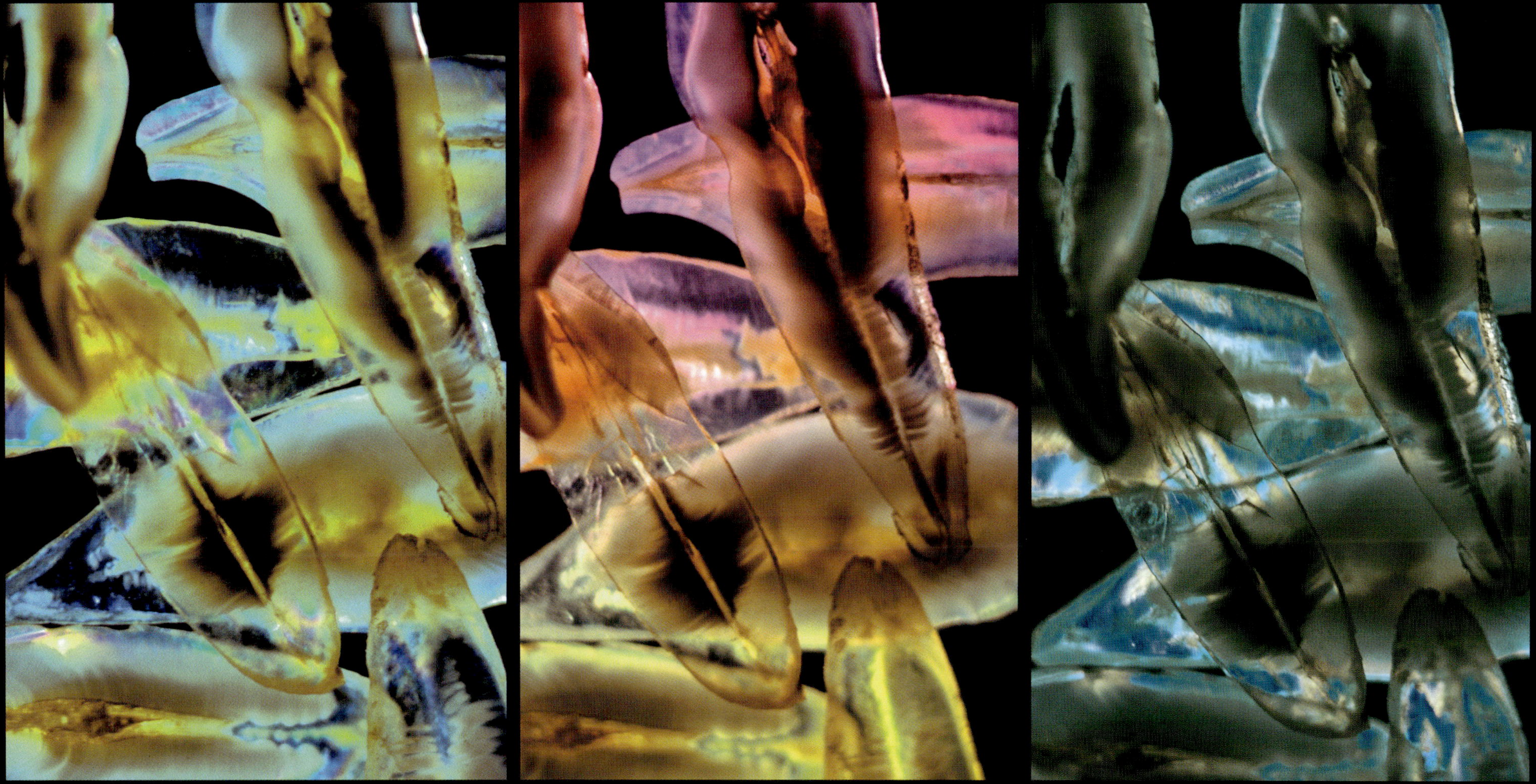

106

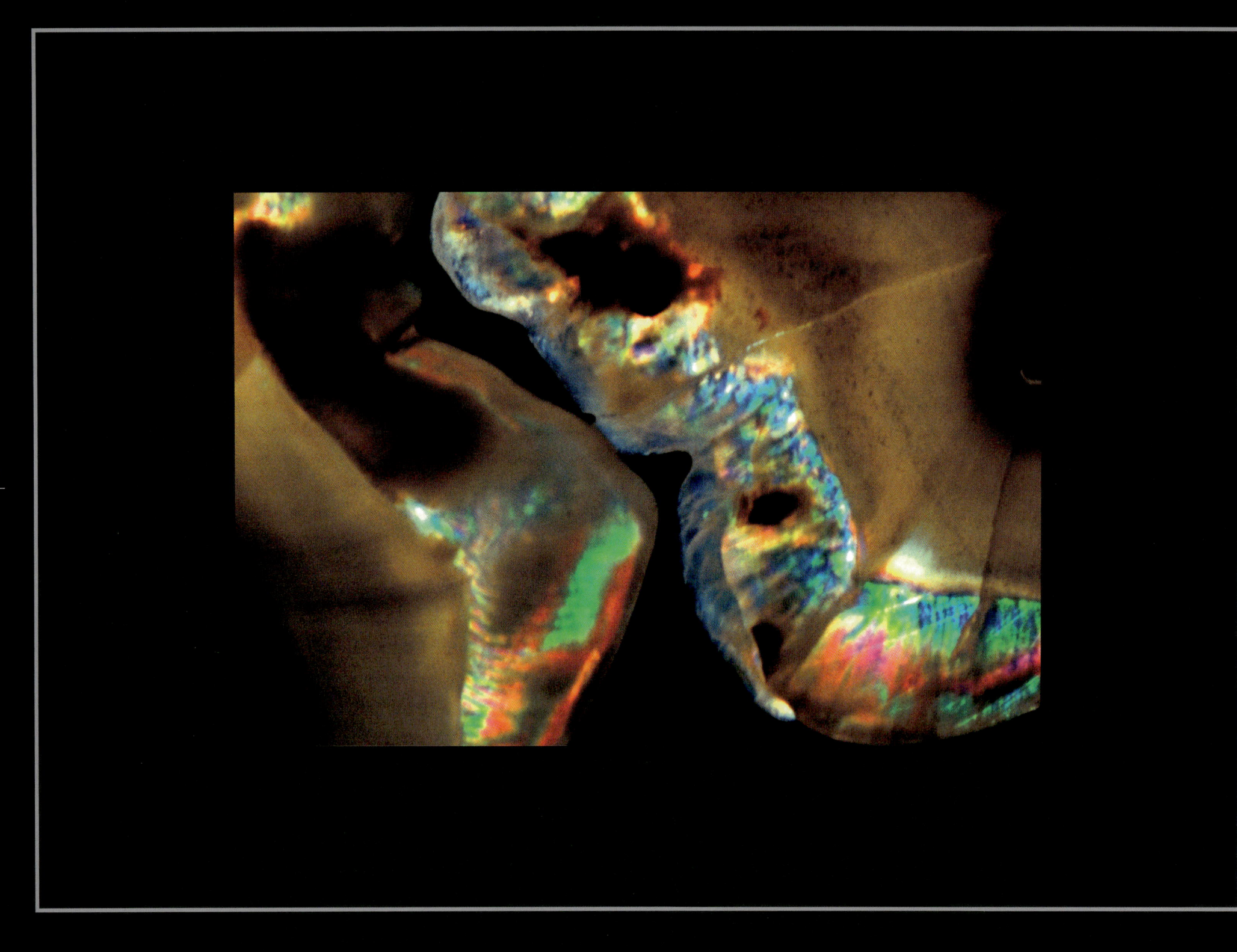

107

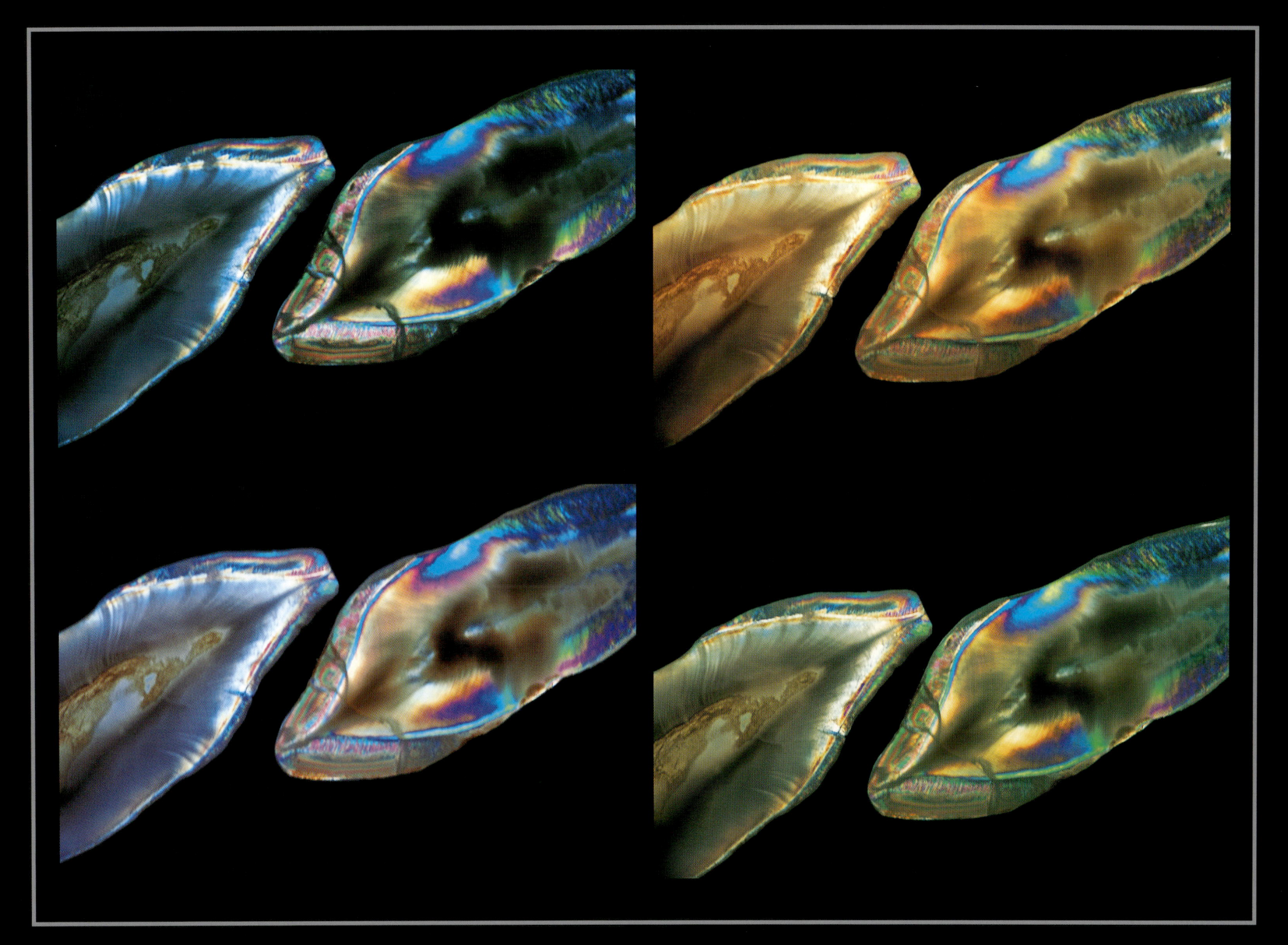

108

109

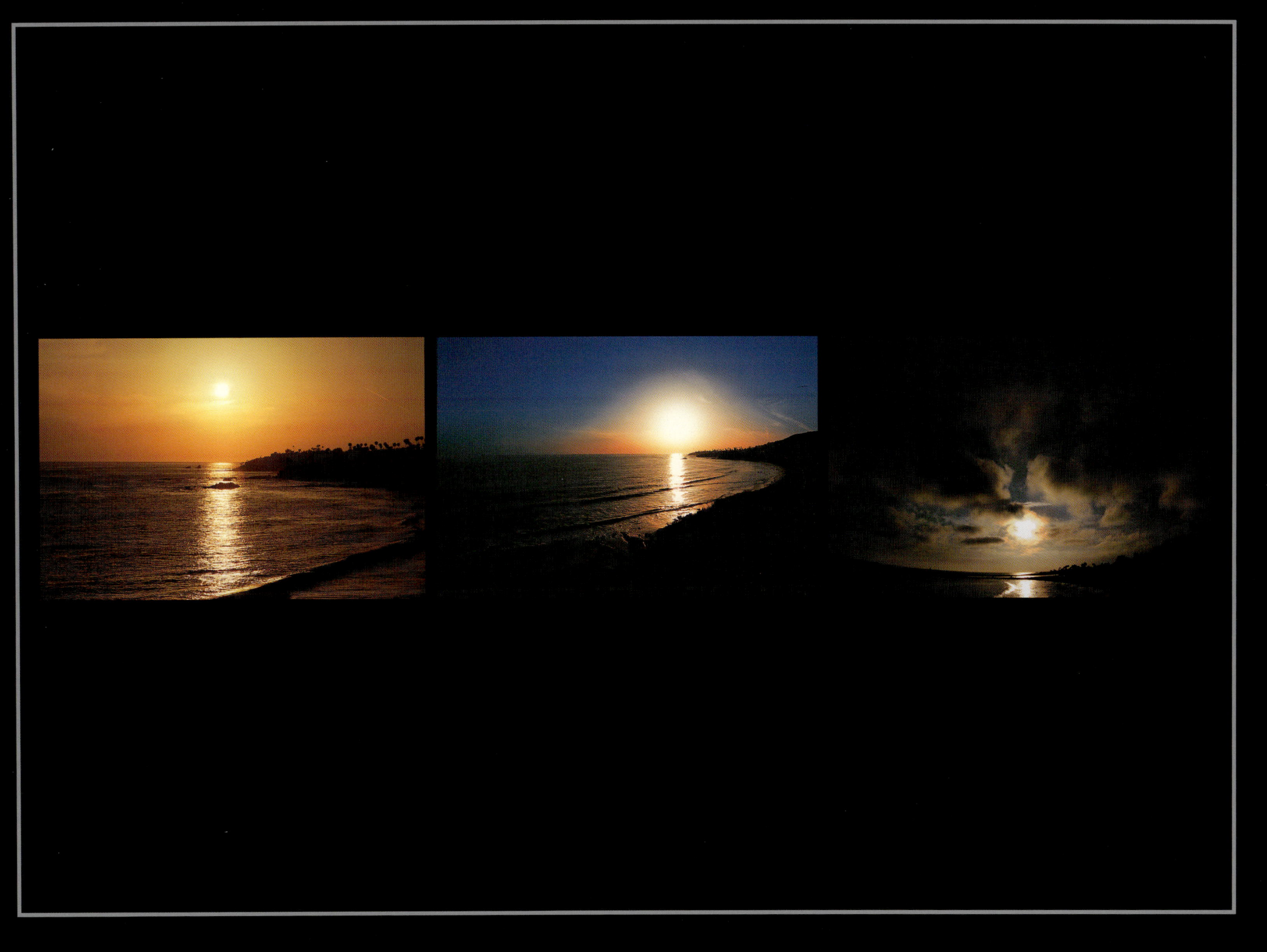

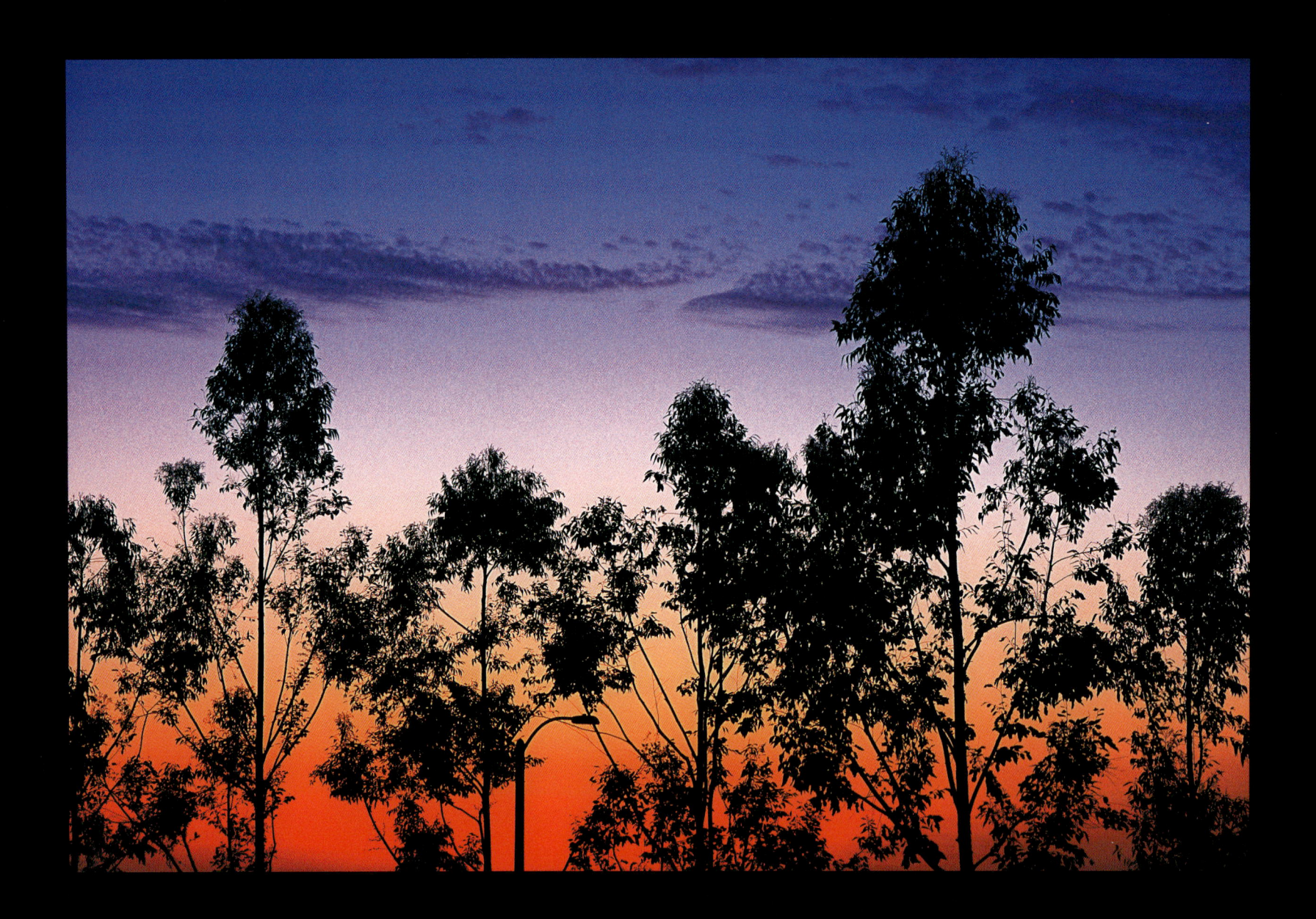

111

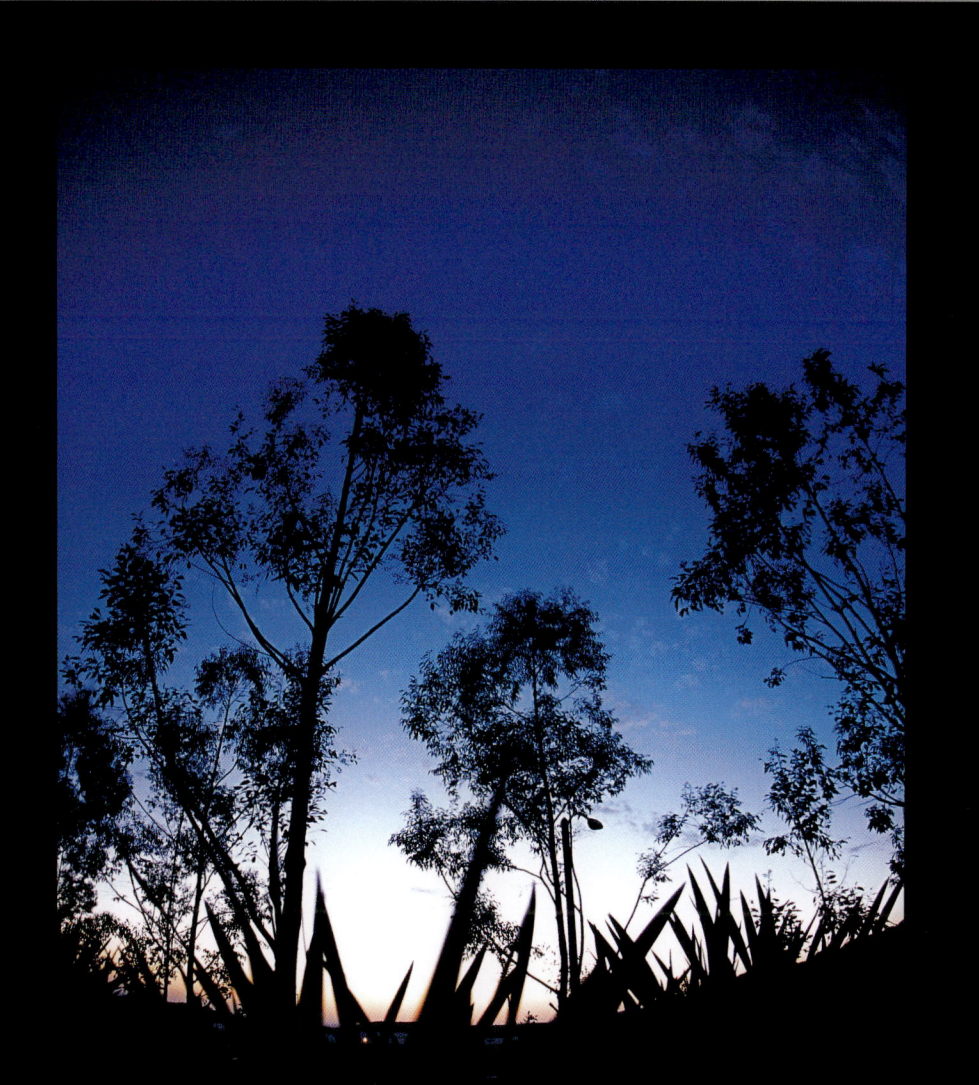

112

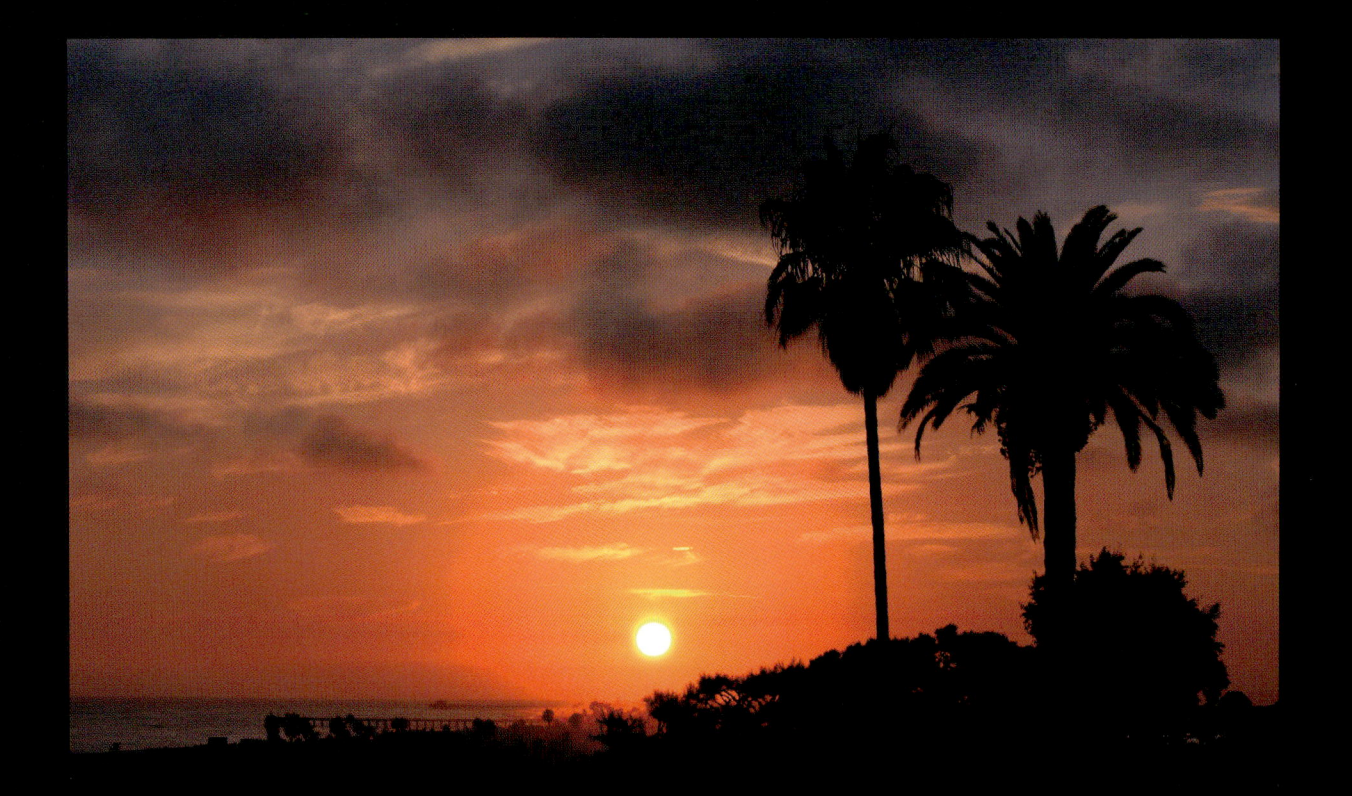

113

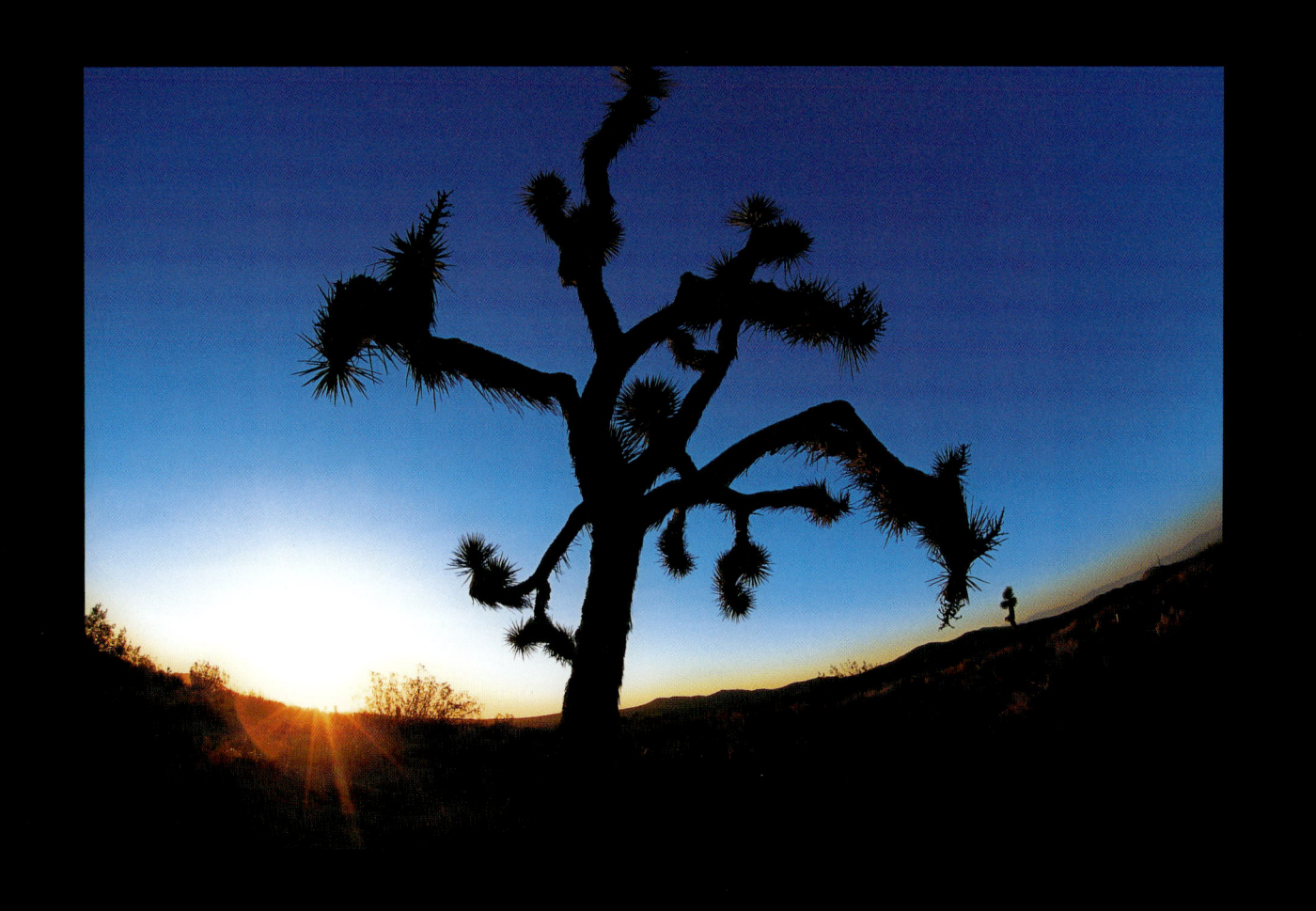

114

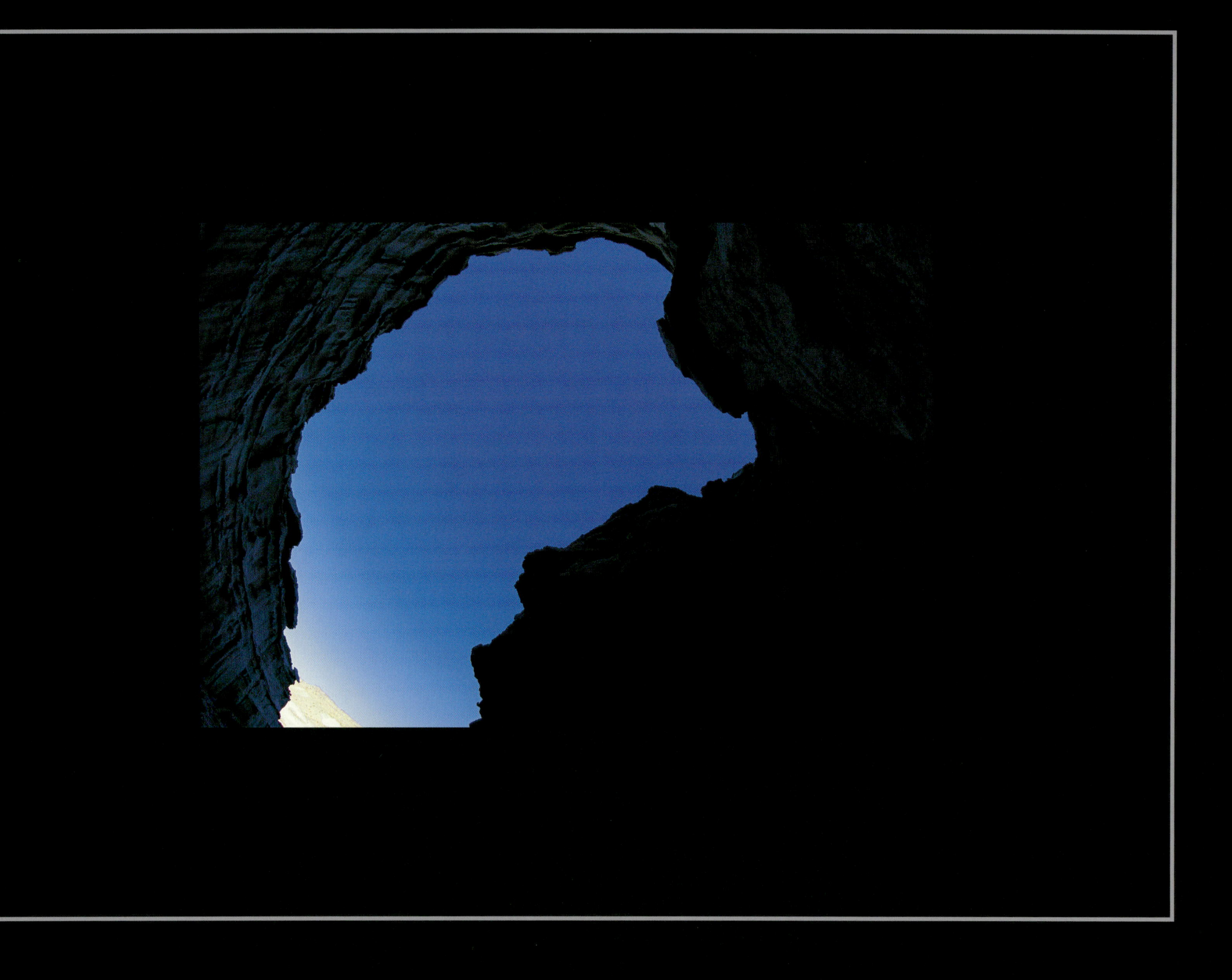

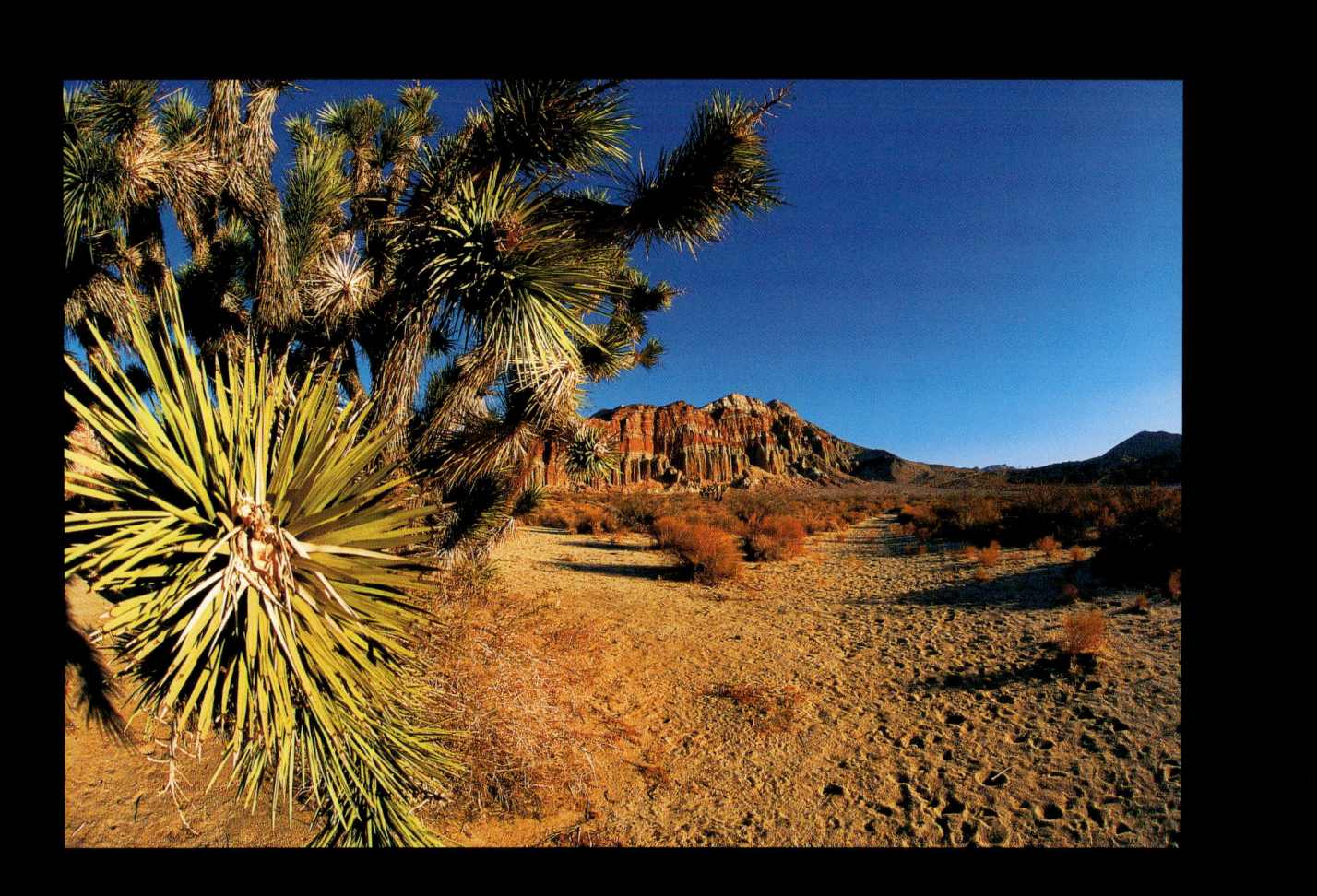

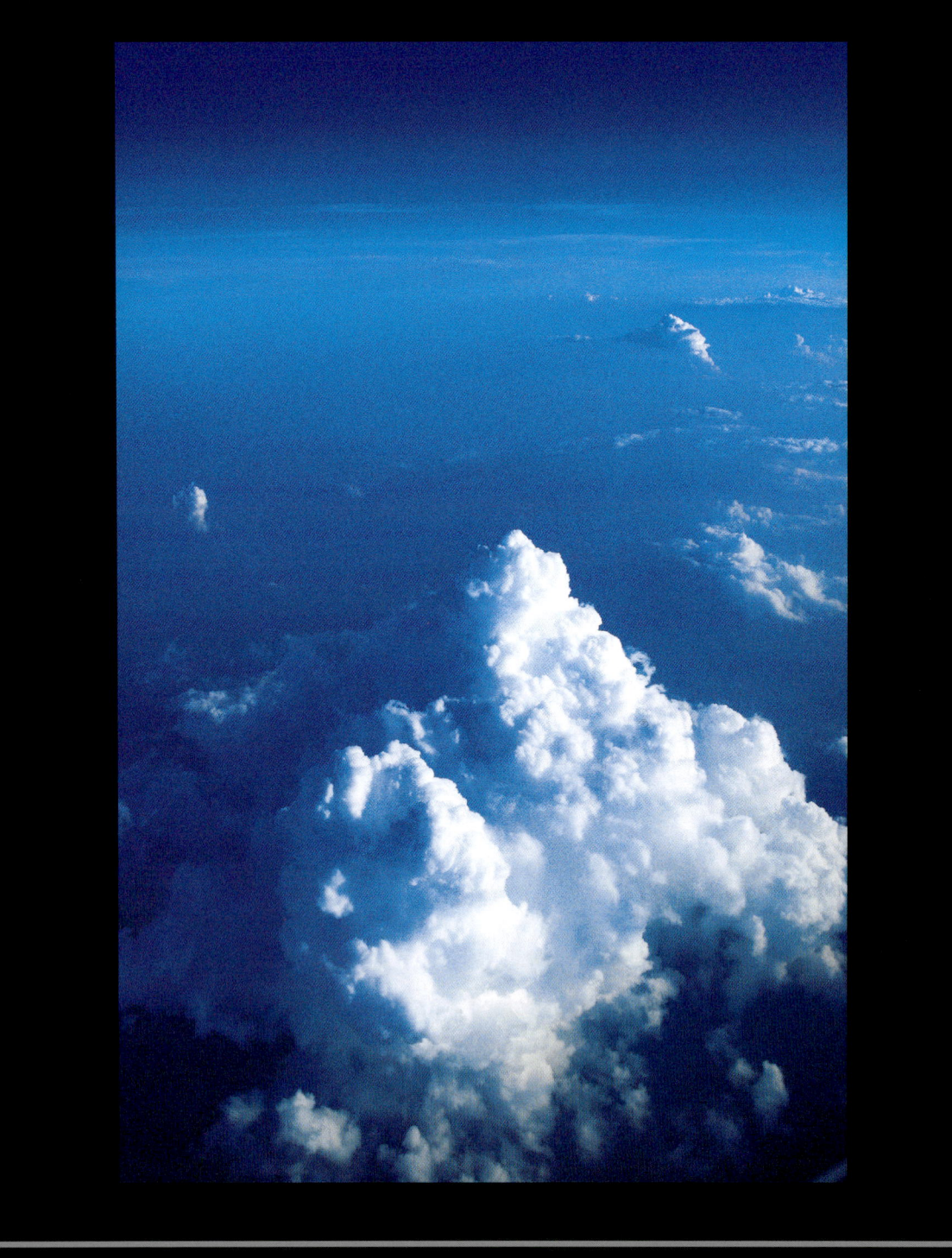

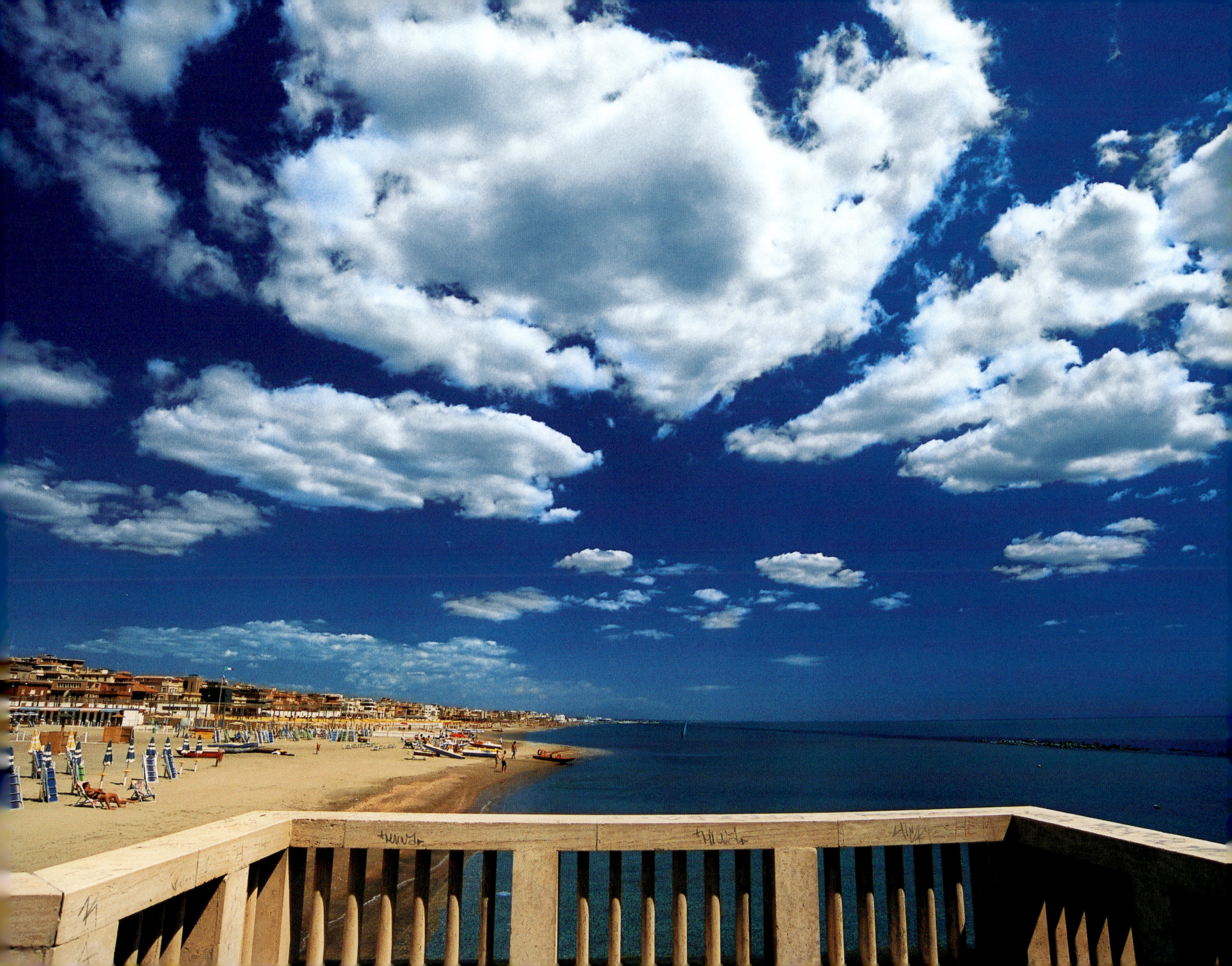

118

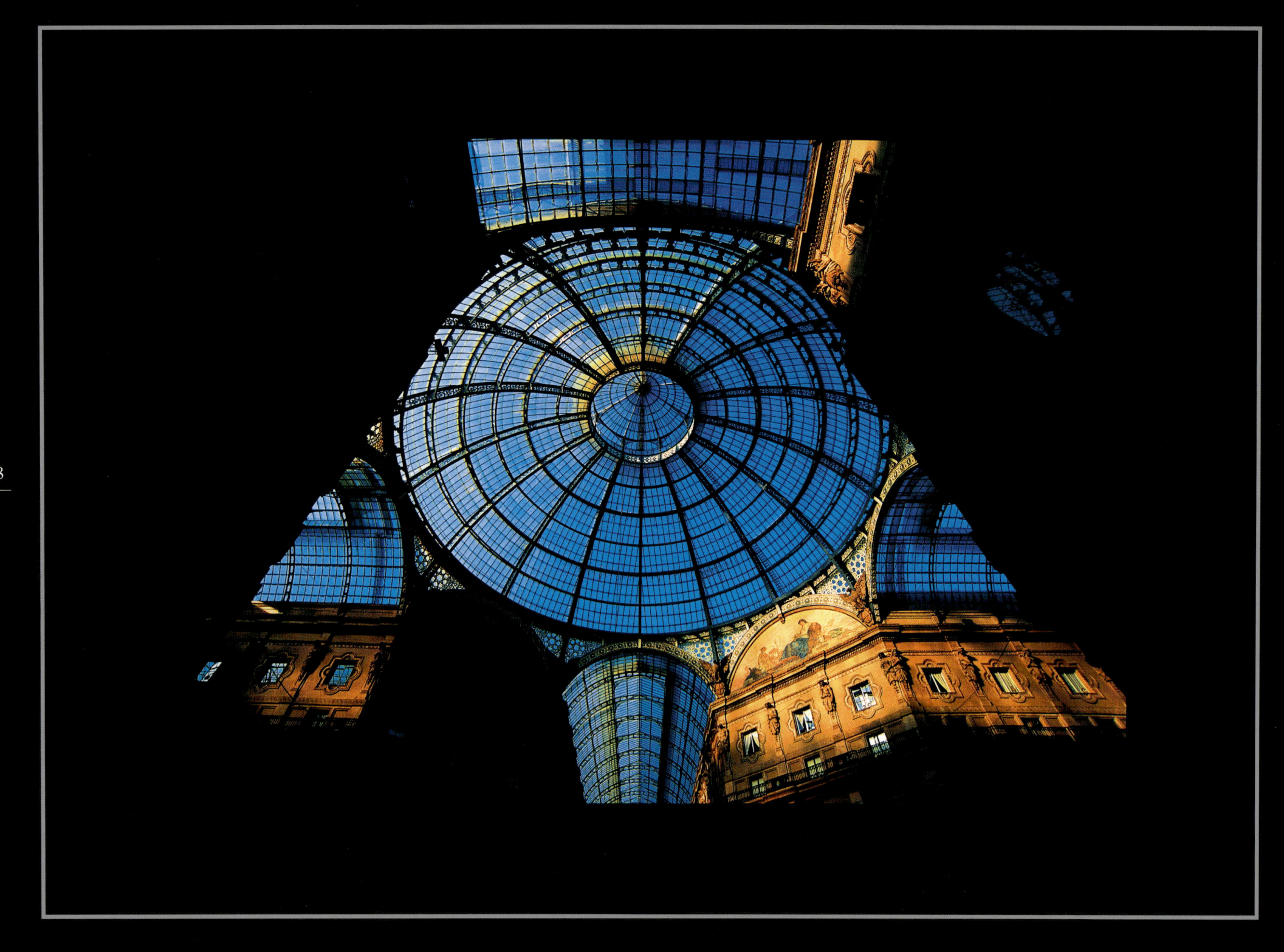

119

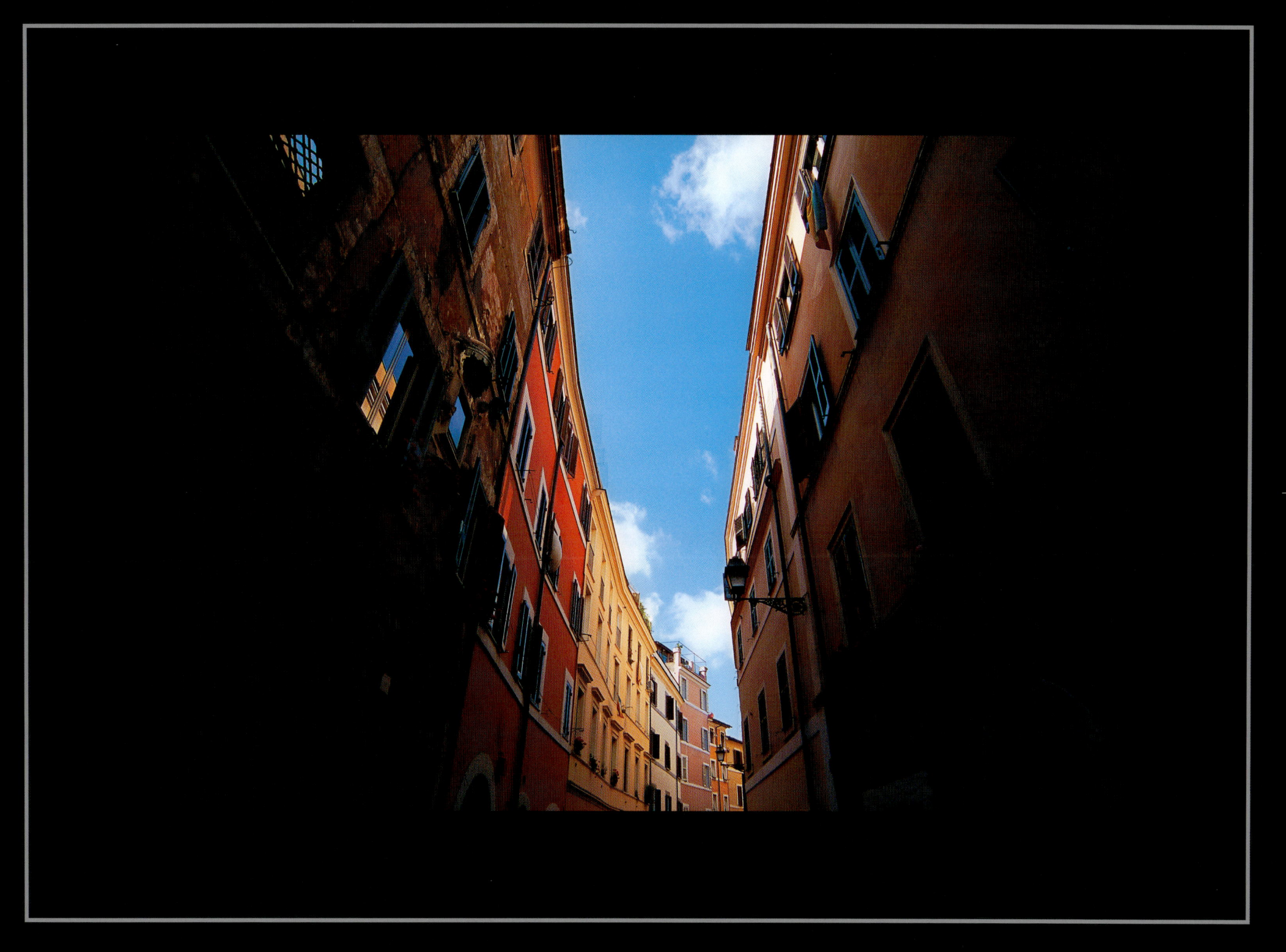

120

121

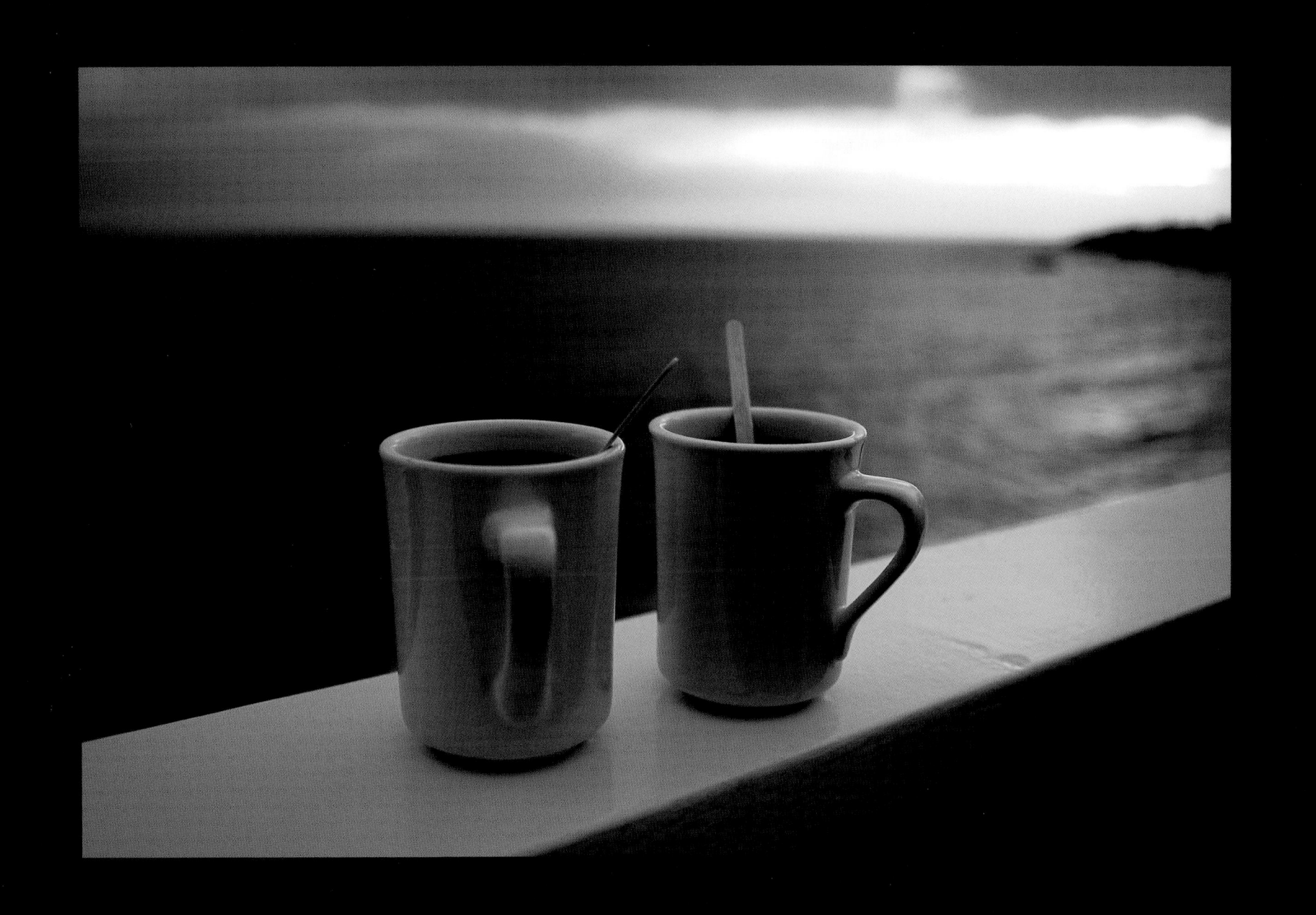

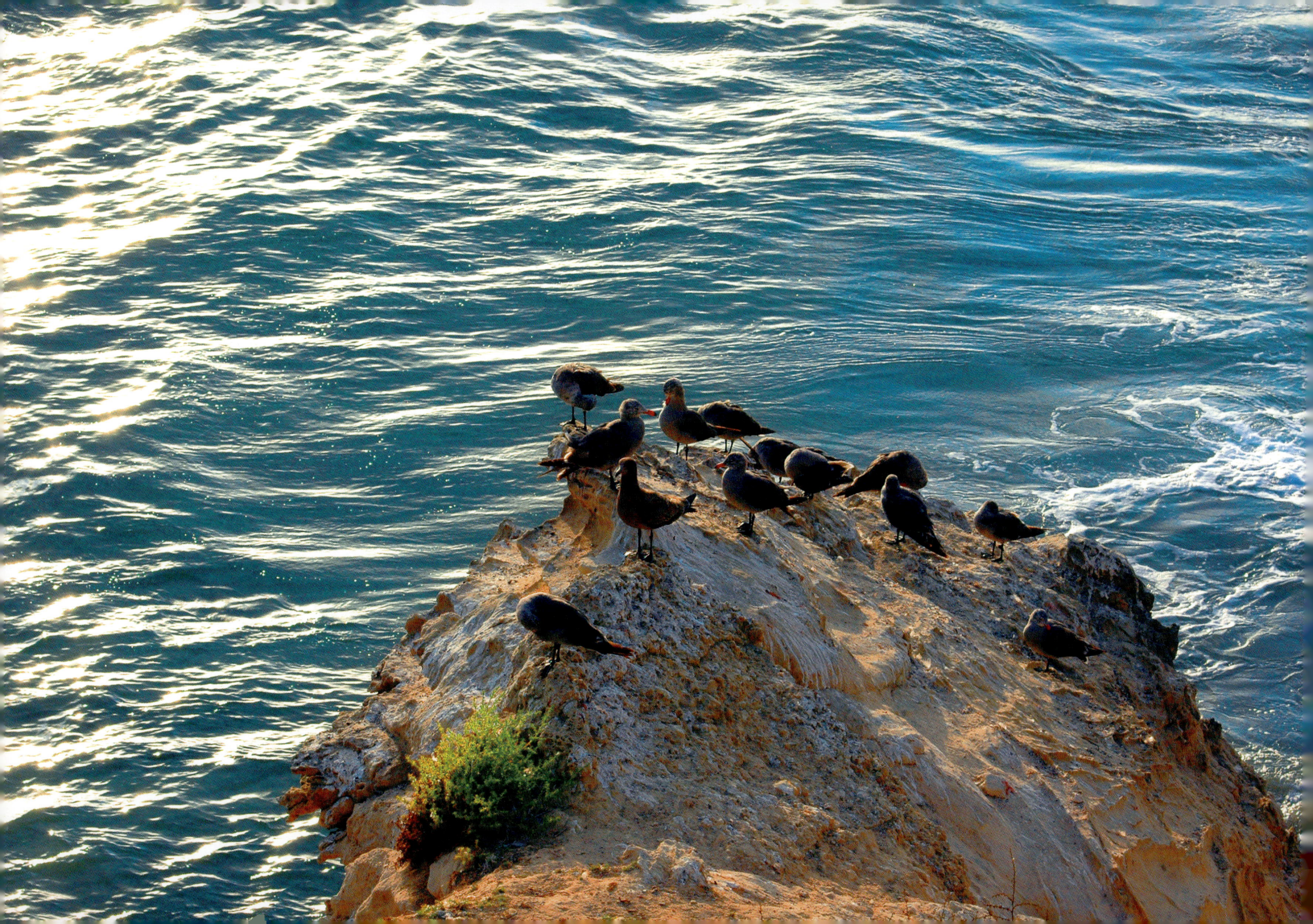

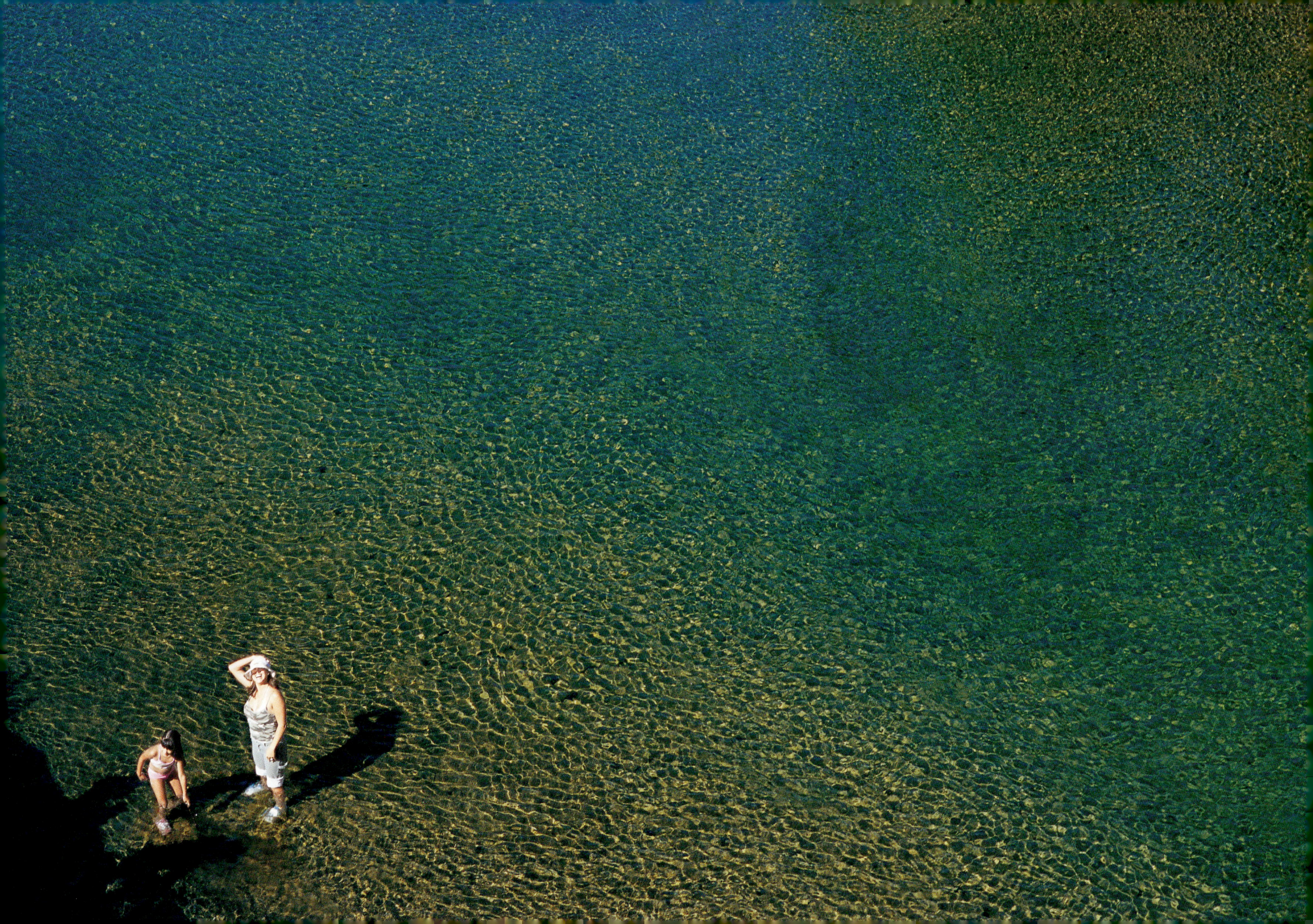

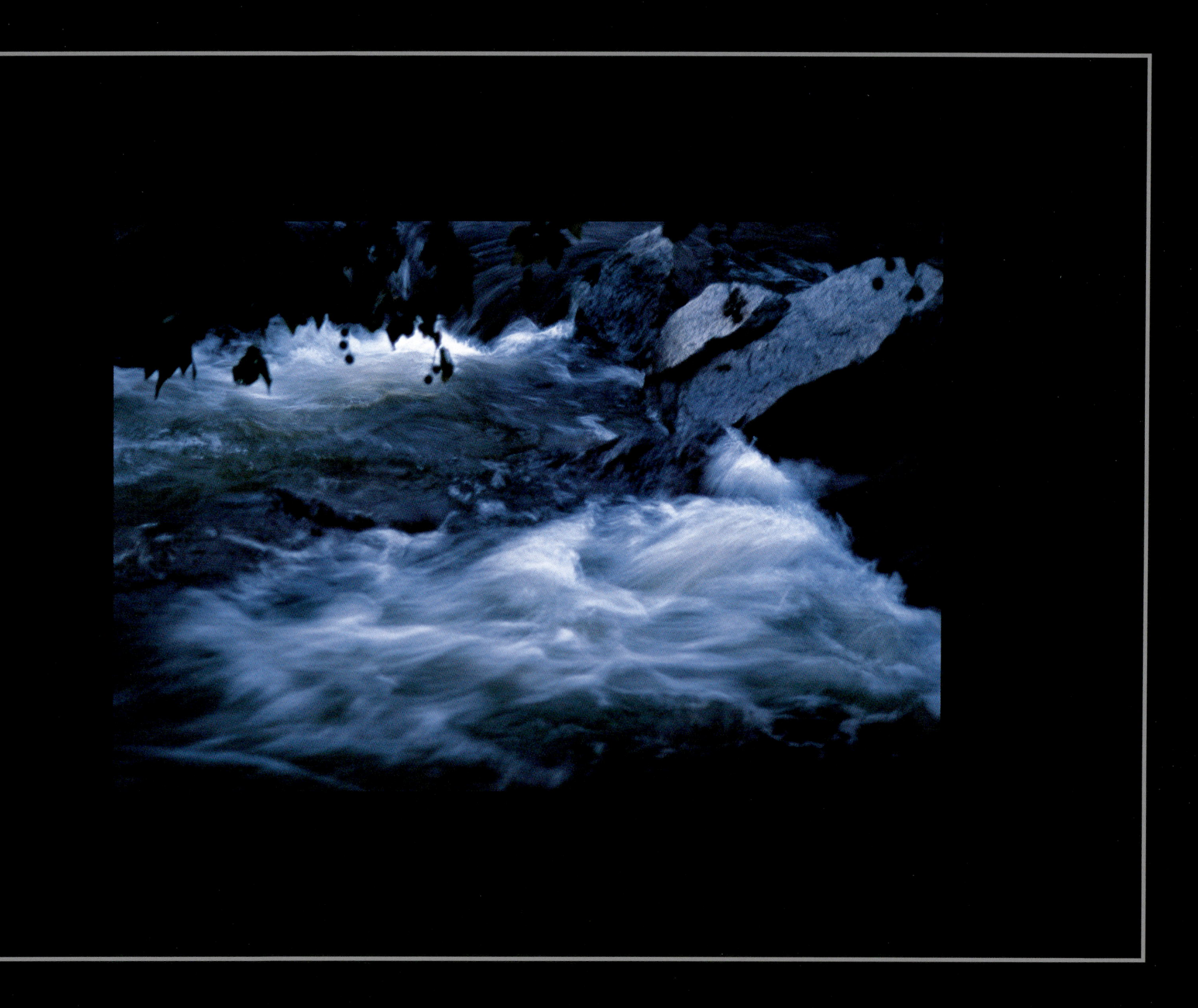

125

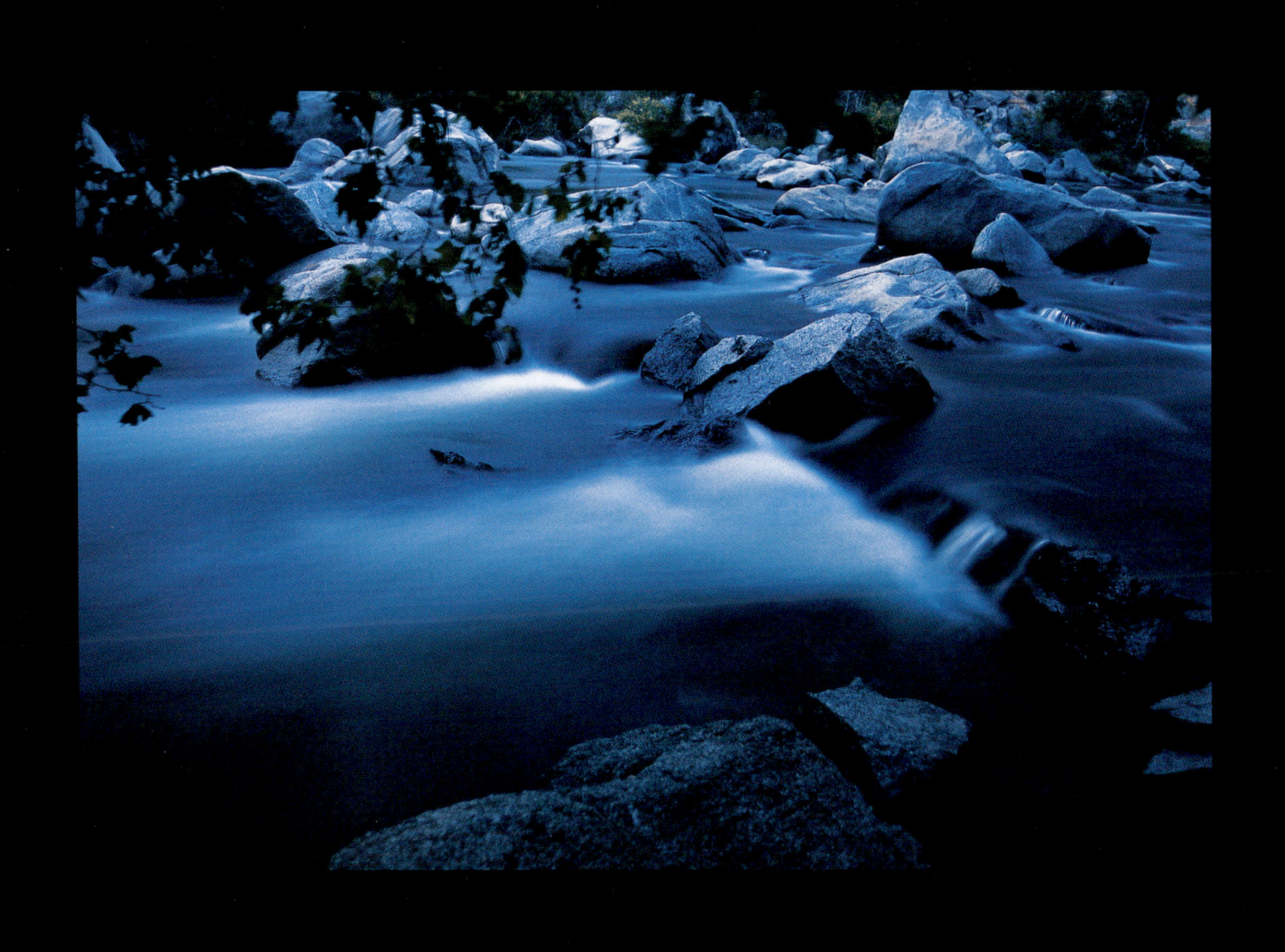

VISION

視野

"The Best Way to See the Future is to Create It"

───創造こそが歩む未来をきりひらく───

127

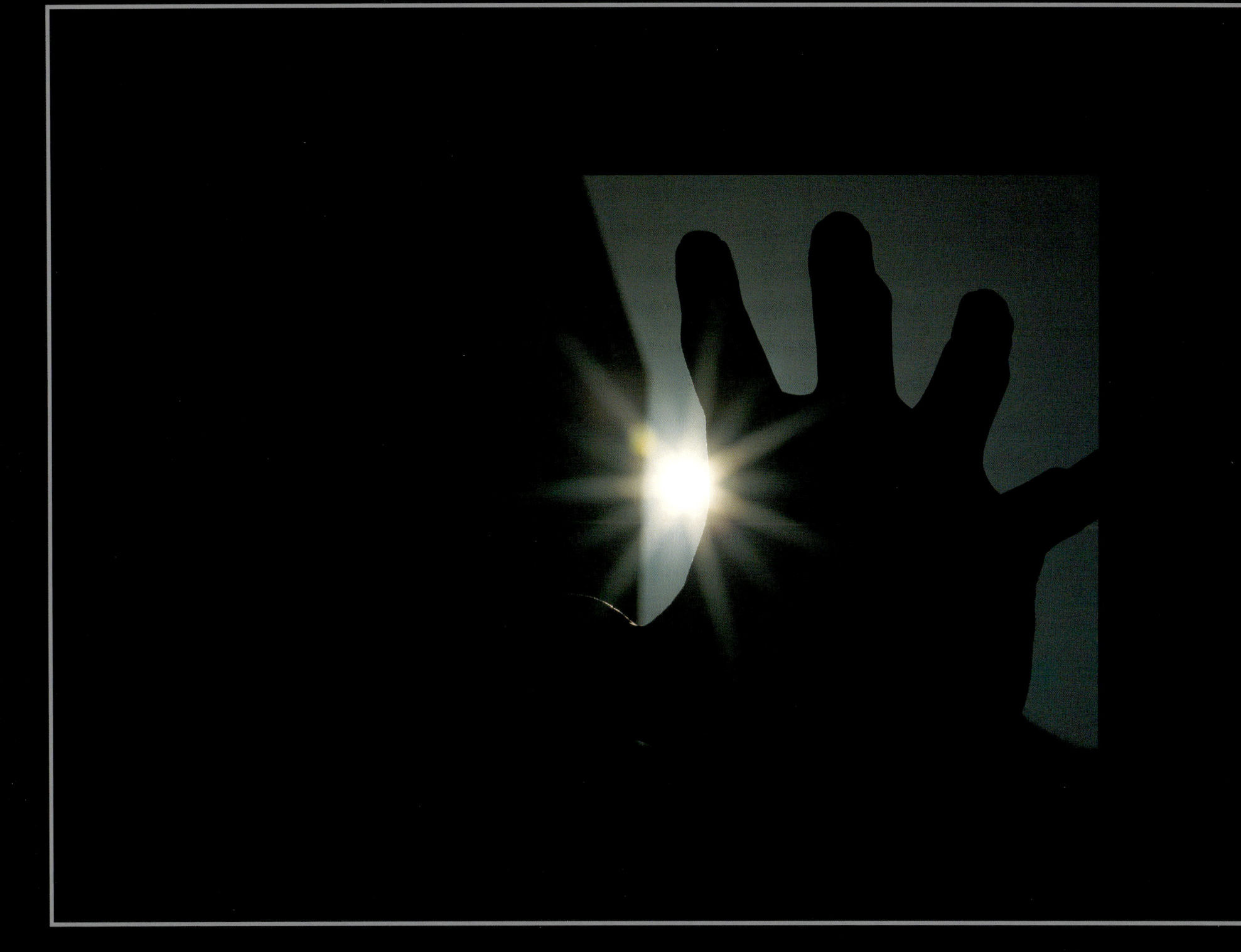

CHALLENGE

挑戦

"Dare to Confront What Can Only be Imagined"

――想像し得る可能性に挑み立ち向かう――

129

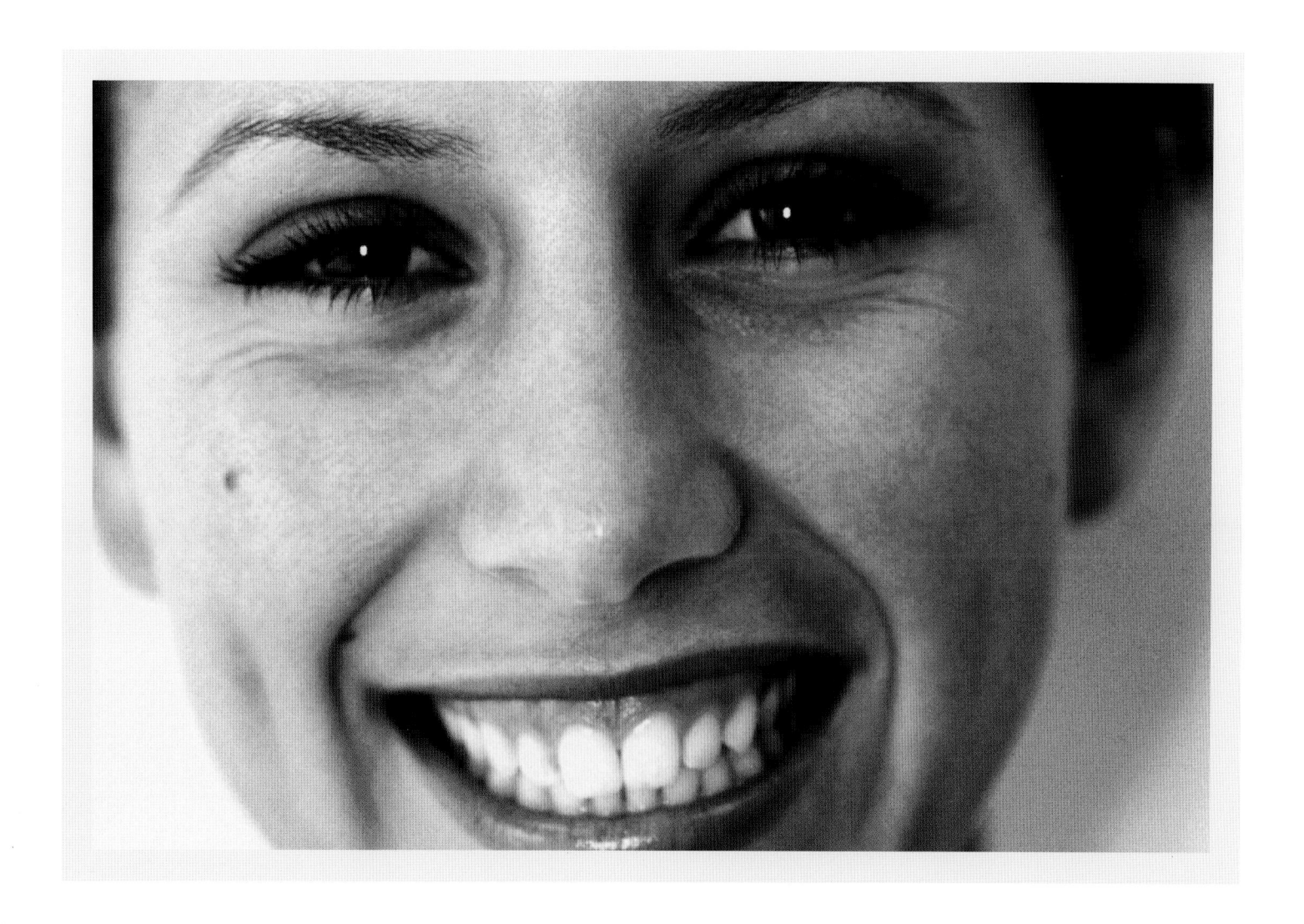

ACHIEVEMENT

達成

"Aim High and Achieve Greatness"

──誇り高き志は偉大な達成へ導く──

131

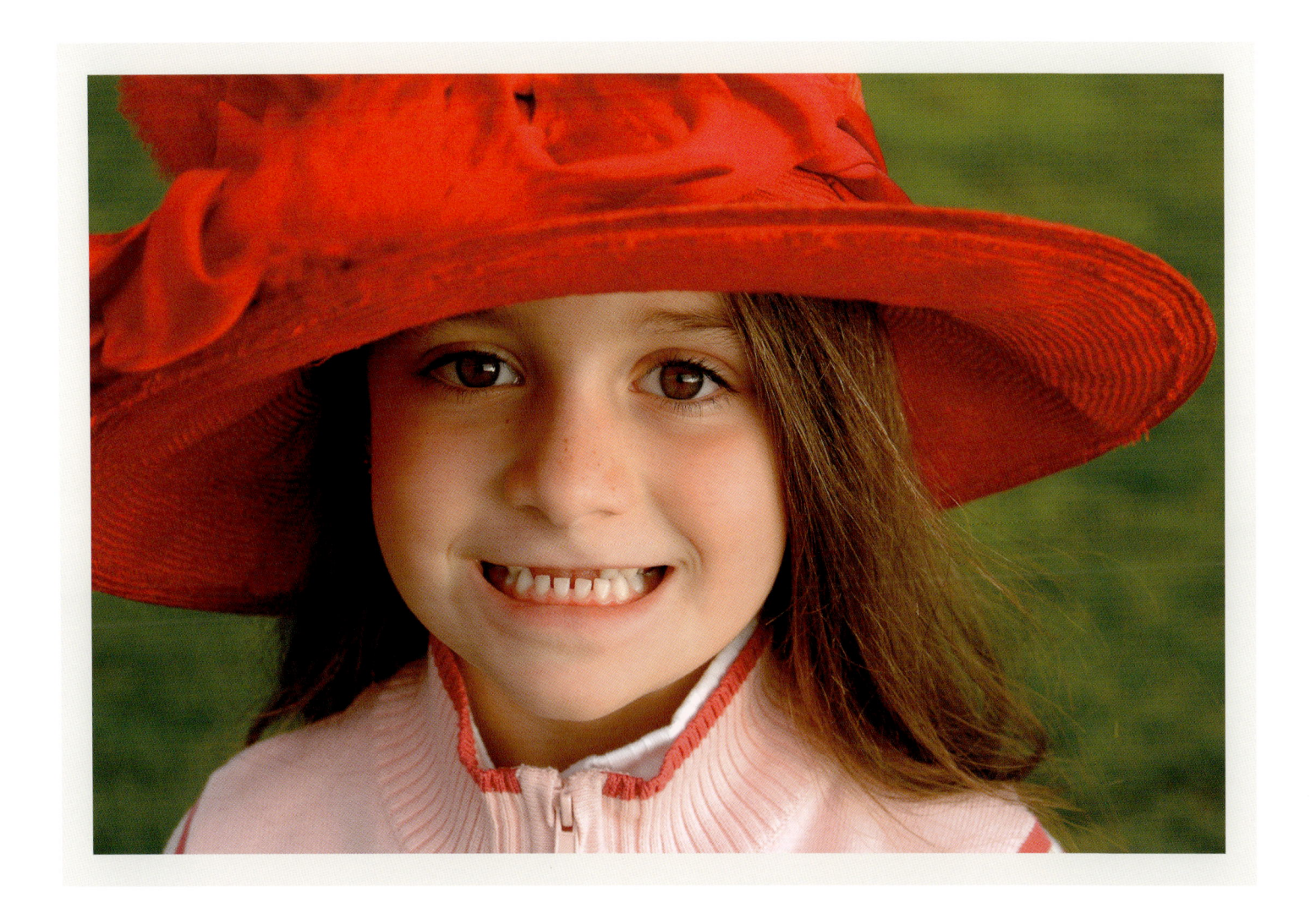

132

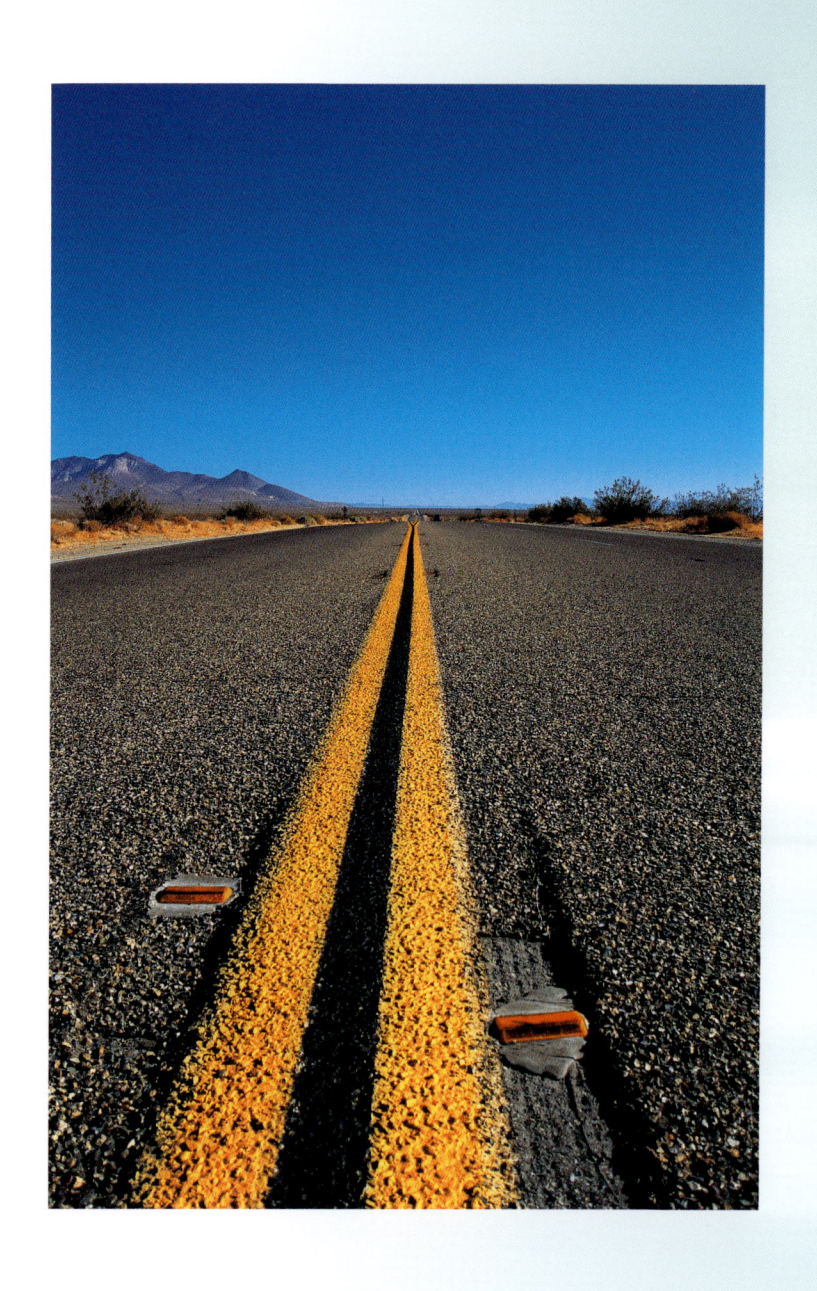

FOLLOW YOUR DREAMS 133

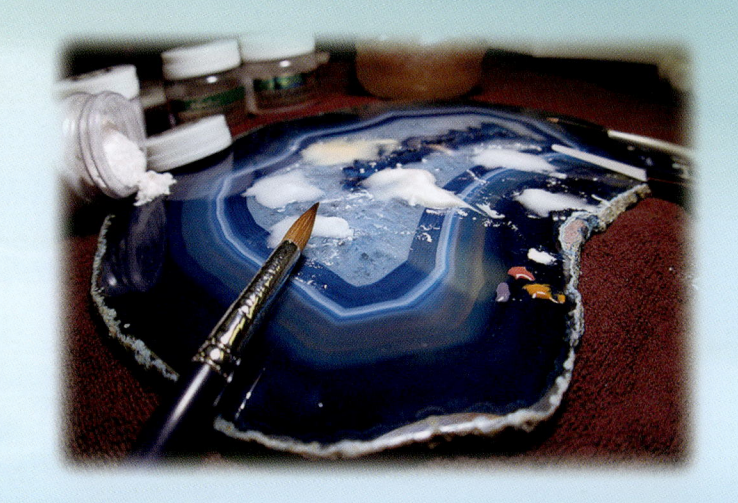

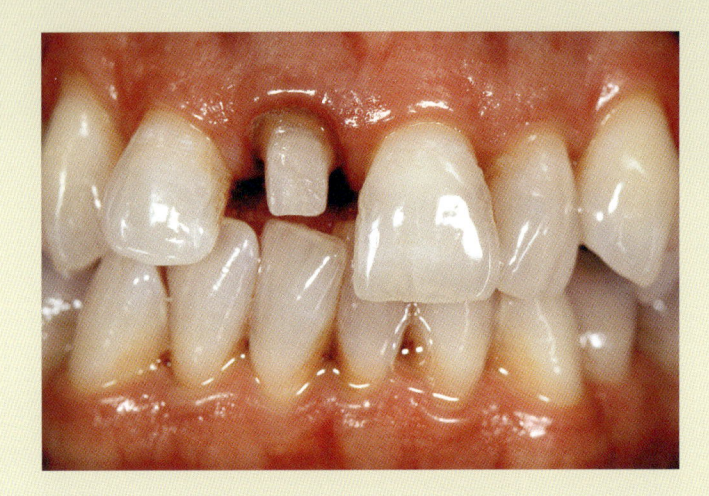

CASE 1 (26-29 page)
メタルセラミック・クラウン(ノリタケAAA陶材使用)。
EX-3 PFM Crown.

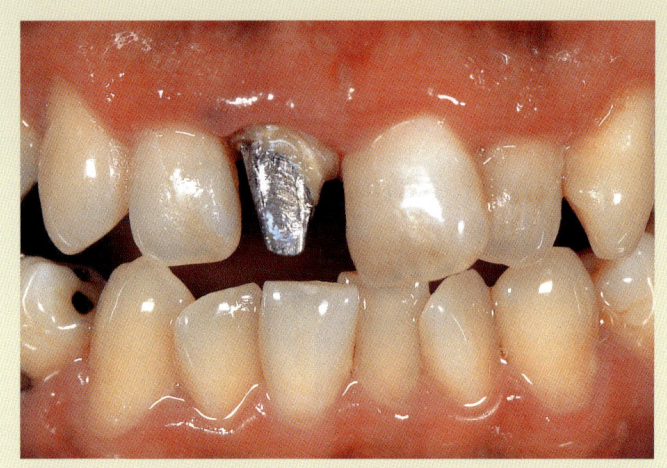

CASE 2 (30 page)
メタルセラミック・クラウン(ノリタケAAA陶材使用)。
EX-3 PFM Crown.

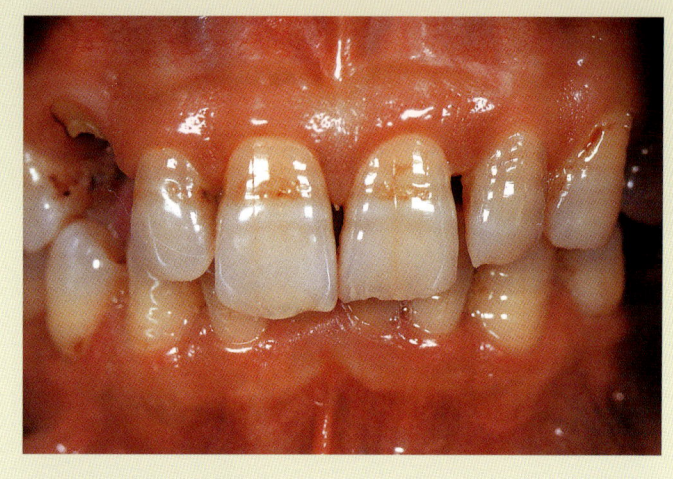

CASE 3 (31 page)
メタルセラミック・クラウン(ノリタケAAA陶材使用)。
EX-3 PFM Crown.

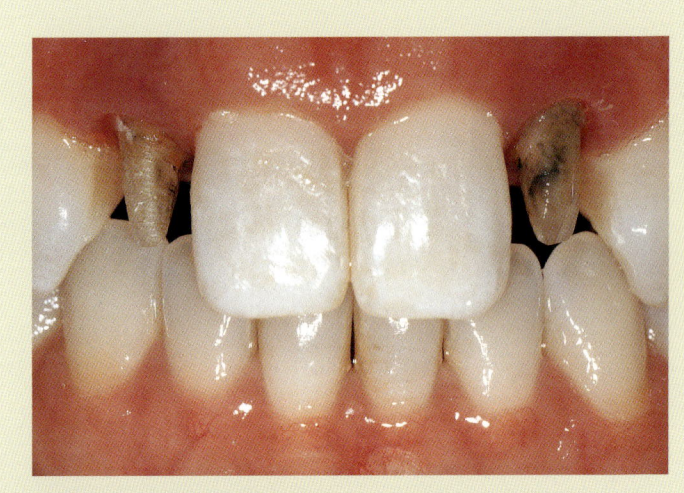

CASE 4 (32-33 page)
メタルセラミック・クラウン(ノリタケAAA陶材使用)。
EX-3 PFM Crown.

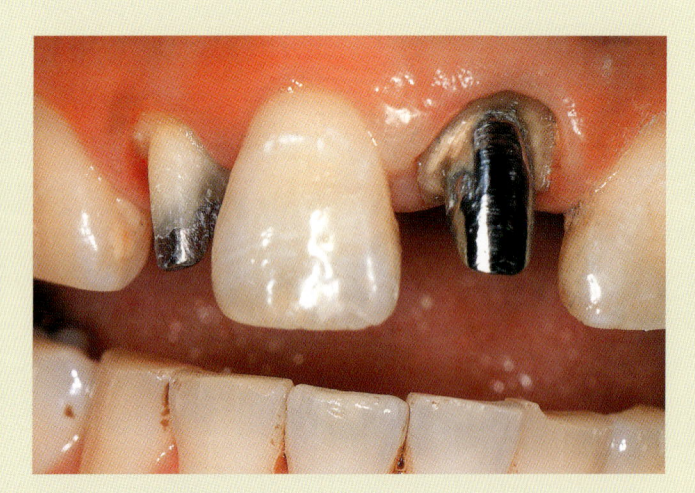

CASE 5 (34-35 page)
メタルセラミック・クラウン(ノリタケAAA陶材使用)。
EX-3 PFM Crown.

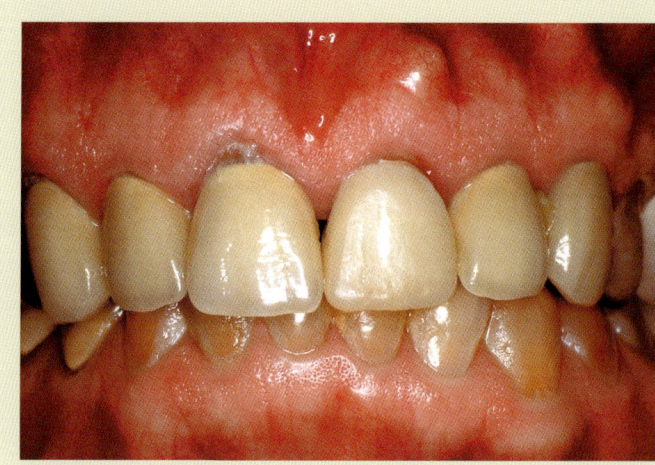

CASE 6 (36-37 page)
メタルセラミック・クラウン(ノリタケAAA陶材使用)。
EX-3 PFM Crown.

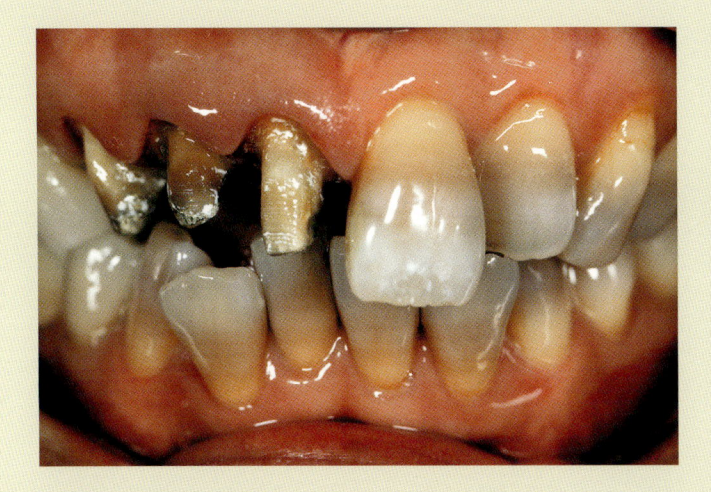

CASE 7　(38-40 page)
メタルセラミック・クラウン(ノリタケAAA陶材使用)。
EX-3 PFM Crown.

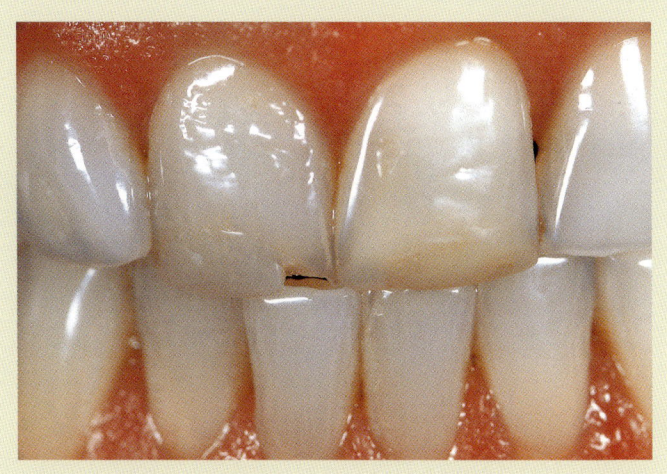

CASE 8　(42-45 page)
PROCERAジルコニア・クラウン(ノリタケCZR陶材使用)。
CZR with PROCERA Zirconia.

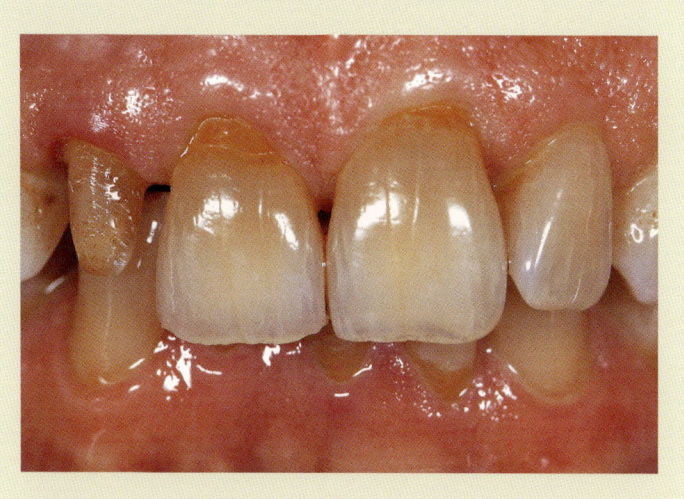

CASE 9　(46-47 page)
PROCERAジルコニア・クラウン(ノリタケCZR陶材使用)。
CZR with PROCERA Zirconia.

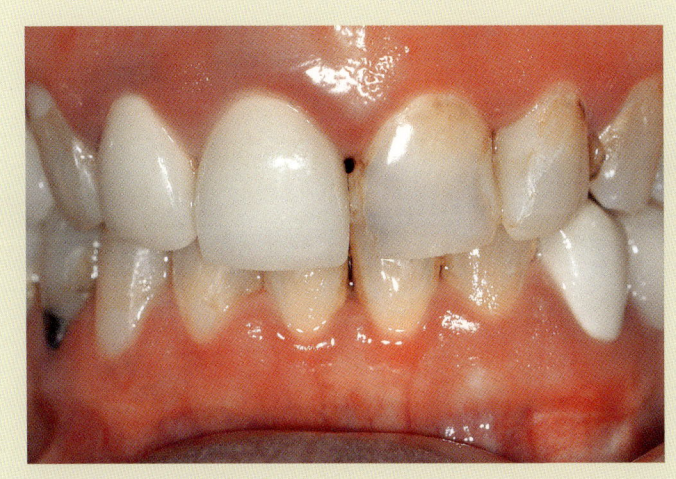

CASE 10　(48 page)
PROCERAジルコニア・クラウン(ノリタケCZR陶材使用)。
CZR with PROCERA Zirconia.

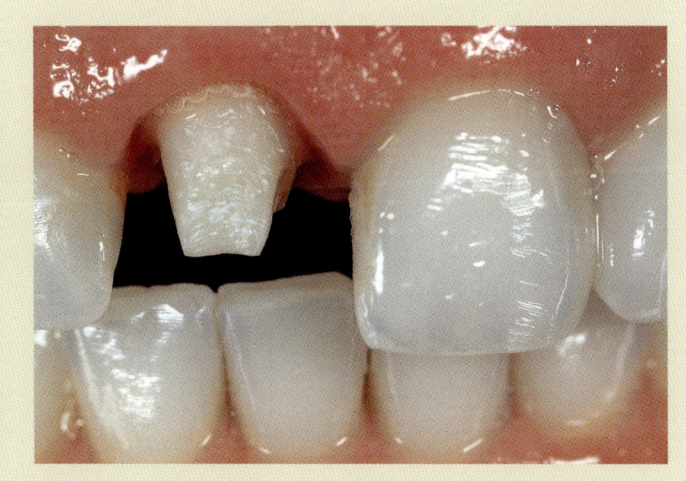

CASE 11　(49 page)
PROCERAジルコニア・クラウン(ノリタケCZR陶材使用)。
CZR with PROCERA Zirconia.

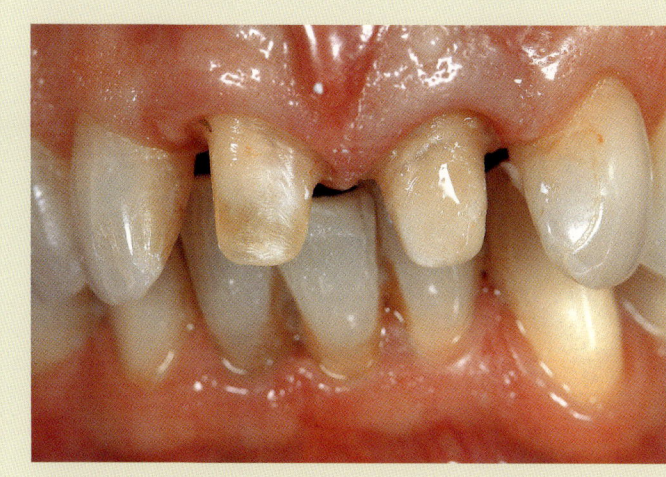

CASE 12　(50 page)
PROCERAジルコニア・クラウン(ノリタケCZR陶材使用)。
CZR with PROCERA Zirconia.

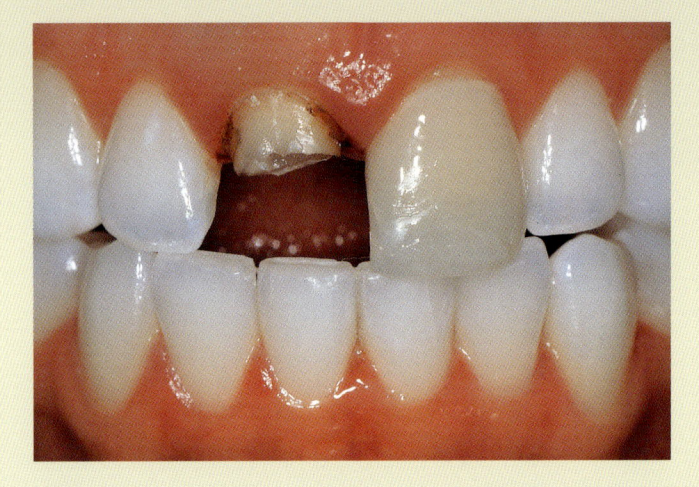

CASE 13　(51 page)
PROCERAジルコニア・クラウン(ノリタケCZR陶材使用)。
CZR with PROCERA Zirconia.

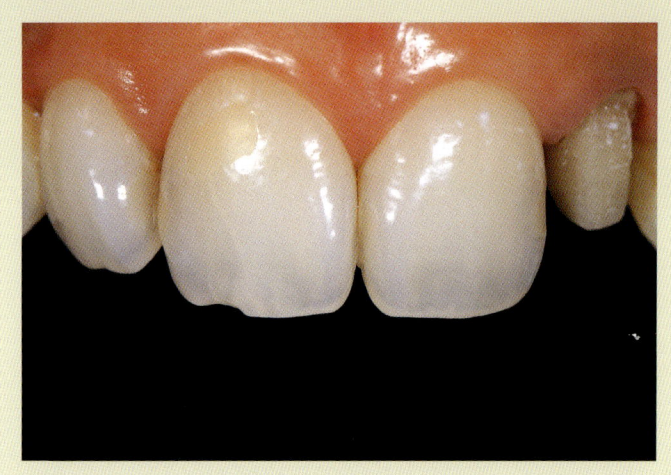

CASE 14　(52-53 page)
PROCERAジルコニア・クラウン(ノリタケCZR陶材使用)。
CZR with PROCERA Zirconia.

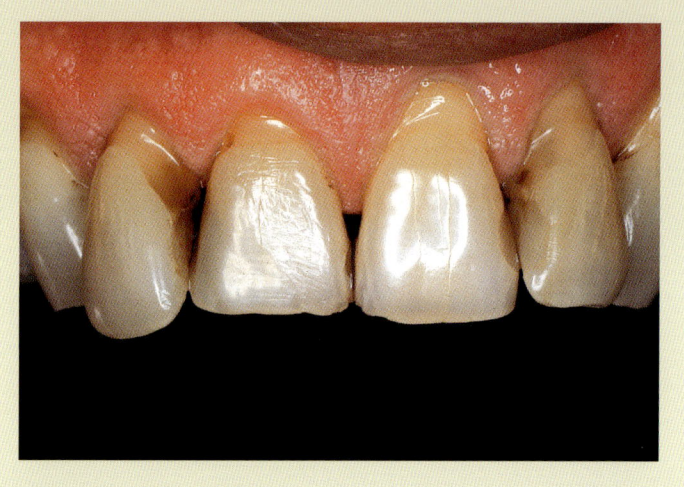

CASE 15　(54 page)
PROCERAアルミナ・クラウン(ノリタケCERABIEN陶材使用)。
CERABIEN with PROCERA Aluminus.

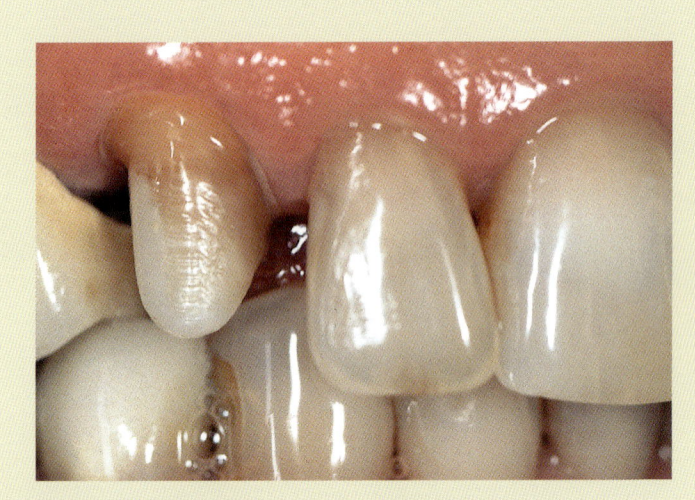

CASE 16　(55 page)
PROCERAアルミナ・クラウン(ノリタケCERABIEN陶材使用)。
CERABIEN with PROCERA Aluminus.

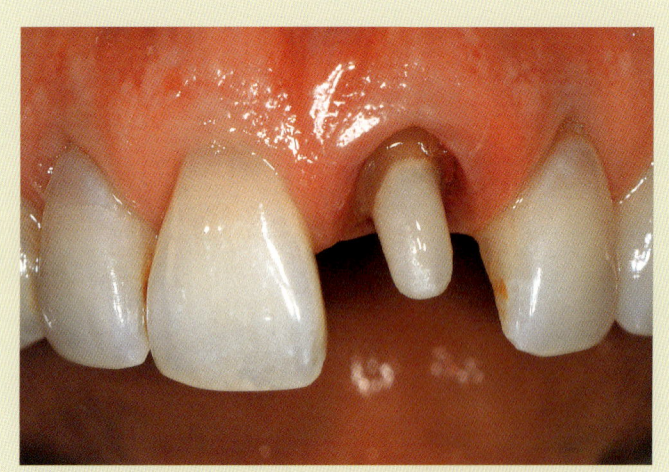

CASE 17　(56-57 page)
PROCERAアルミナ・クラウン(ノリタケCERABIEN陶材使用)。
CERABIEN with PROCERA Aluminus.

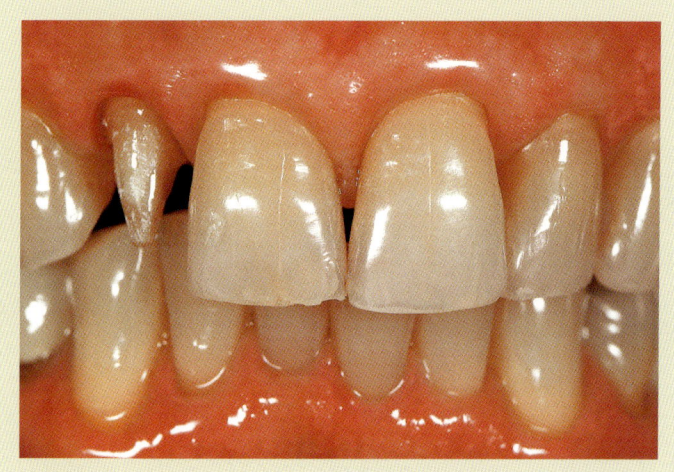

CASE 18　(58 page)
PROCERAアルミナ・クラウン(ノリタケCERABIEN陶材使用)。
CERABIEN with PROCERA Aluminus.

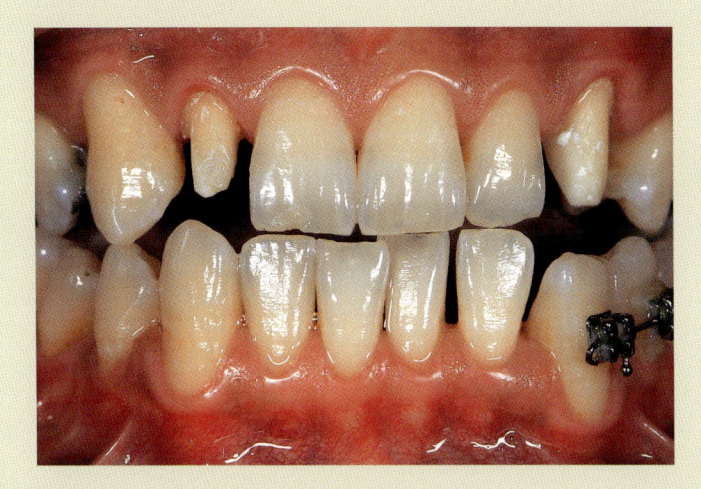

CASE 19 (59 page)
PROCERAアルミナ・クラウン(ノリタケCERABIEN陶材使用)。
CERABIEN with PROCERA Aluminus.

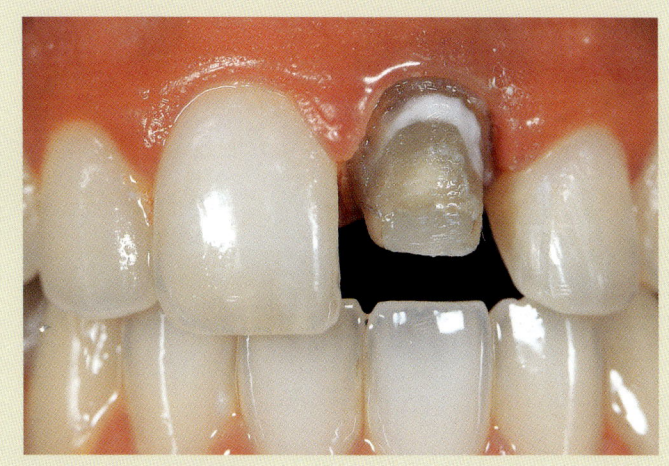

CASE 20 (60 page)
ポーセレン・ジャケットクラウン(ノリタケAAA陶材使用)。
EX-3 Porcelain Jacket Crown.

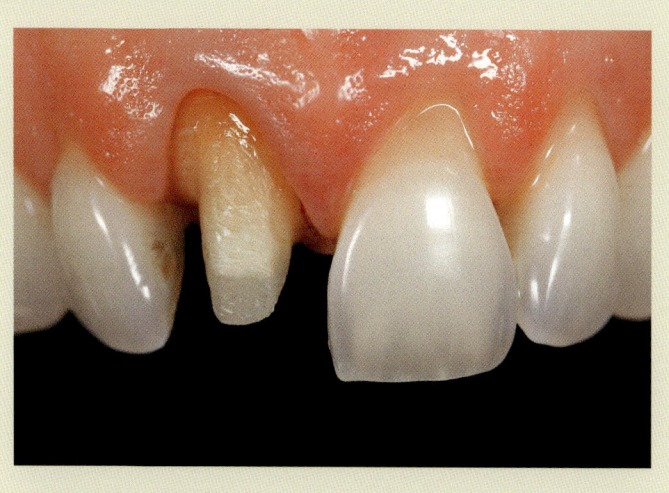

CASE 21 (61 page)
ポーセレン・ジャケットクラウン(ノリタケAAA陶材使用)。
EX-3 Porcelain Jacket Crown.

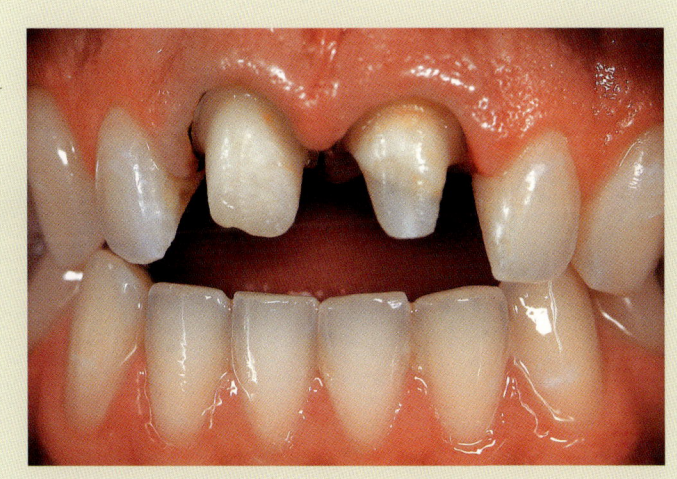

CASE 22 (62 page)
ポーセレン・ジャケットクラウン(ノリタケAAA陶材使用)。
EX-3 Porcelain Jacket Crown.

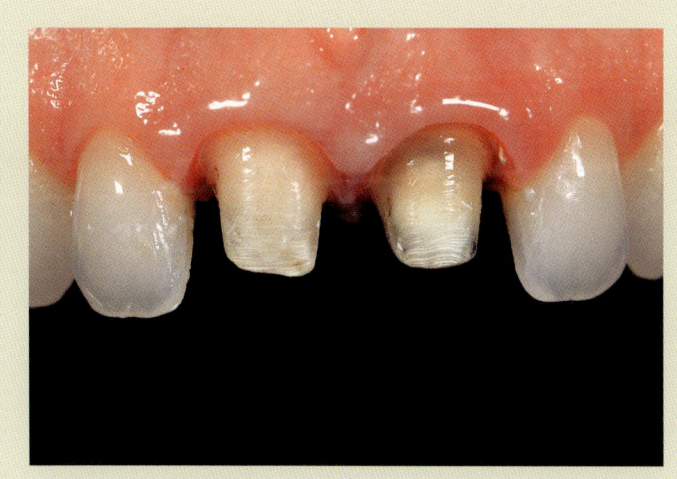

CASE 23 (63 page)
ポーセレン・ジャケットクラウン(ノリタケAAA陶材使用)。
EX-3 Porcelain Jacket Crown.

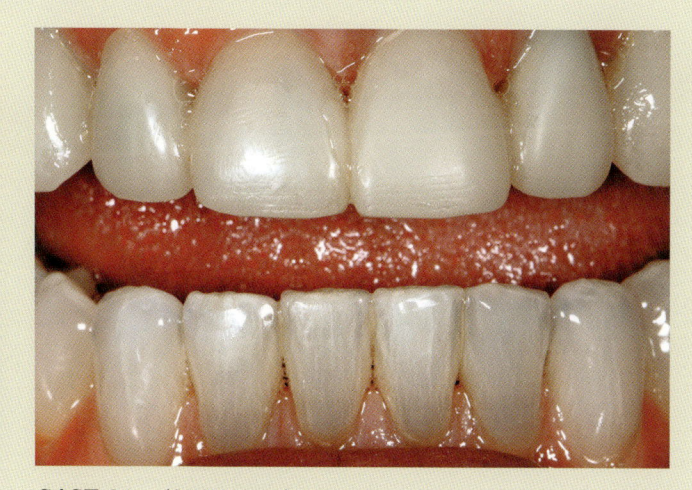

CASE 24 (64-65 page)
ポーセレン・ジャケットクラウン＋
ポーセレンラミネートベニアのコンビネーション(ノリタケAAA陶材使用)。
EX-3 Porcelain Jacket Crown
& Porcelain Laminate Veneers Combination.

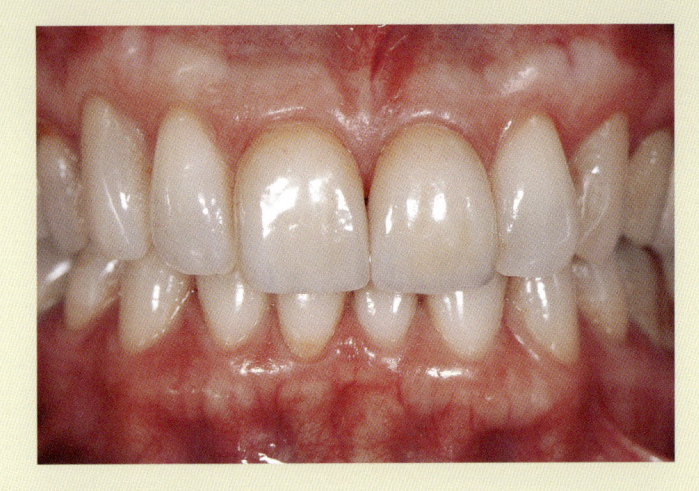

CASE 25 (66-67 page)
ポーセレン・ジャケットクラウン＋ポーセレンラミネートベニアの
コンビネーション(ノリタケAAA陶材使用)。
EX-3 Porcelain Jacket Crown &
Procelain Laminate Veneers Combination.

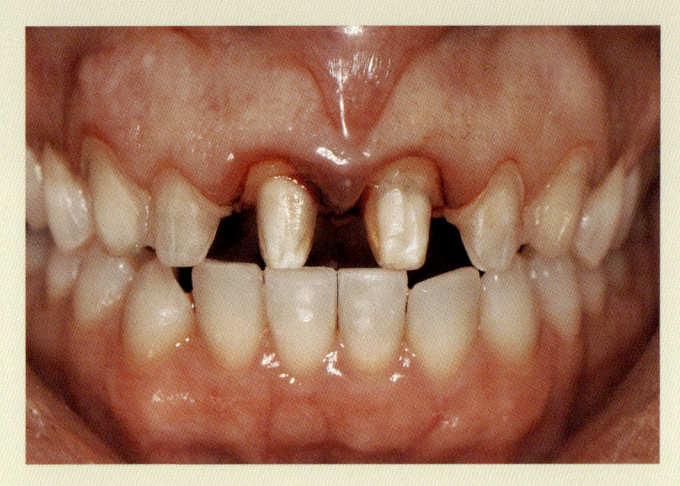

CASE 26 (68 page)
PROCERAアルミナ・クラウン＋ポーセレンラミネートベニアの
コンビネーション(ノリタケCERABIEN, EX-3 陶材使用)。
CERABIEN with PROCERA Aluminus &
Porcelain Laminate Veneers Combination.

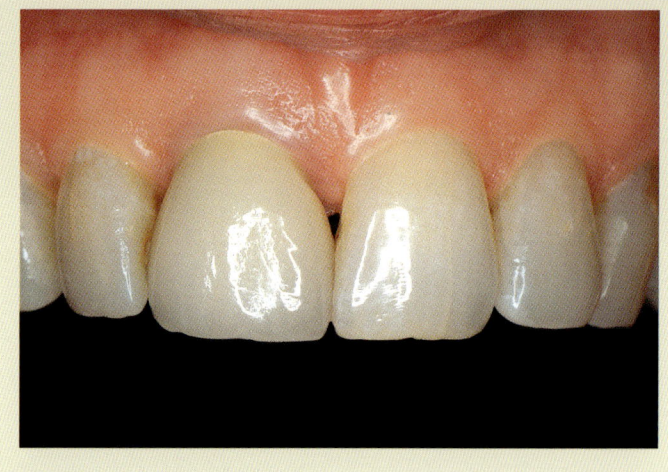

CASE 27 (69 page)
ポーセレン・ジャケットクラウン(ノリタケAAA陶材使用)。
EX-3 Porcelain Jacket Crown.

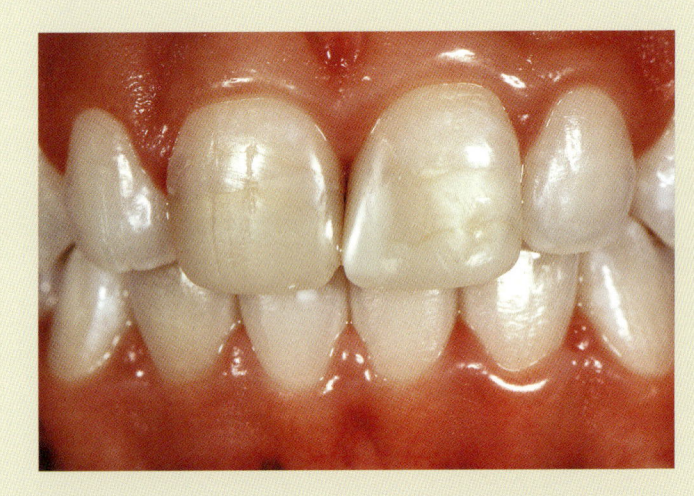

CASE 28 (70-71 page)
ポーセレン・ジャケットクラウン(ノリタケAAA陶材使用)。
EX-3 Porcelain Jacket Crown.

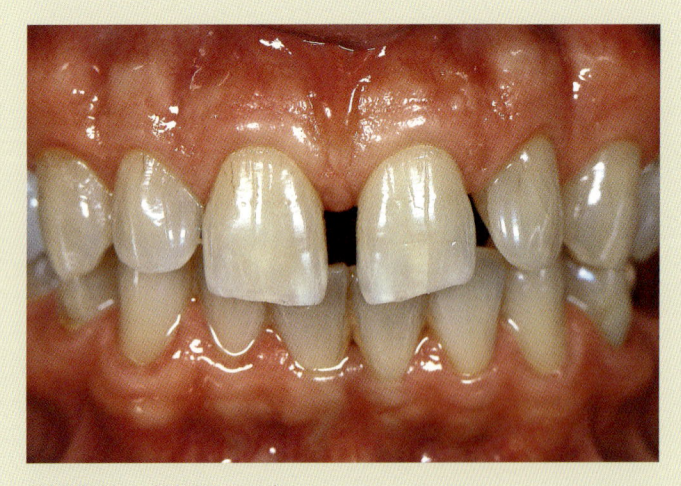

CASE 29 (73-77 page)
ポーセレンラミネートベニア(ノリタケAAA陶材使用)。
EX-3 Porcelain Laminate Veneer.

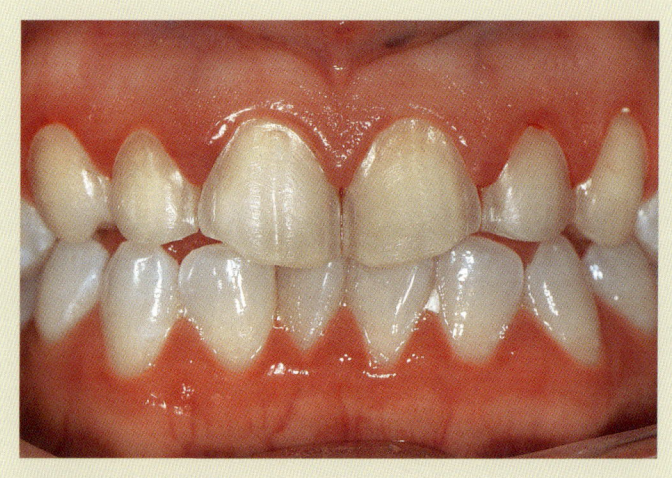

CASE 30 (78-79 page)
ポーセレンラミネートベニア(ノリタケAAA陶材使用)。
EX-3 Porcelain Laminate Veneer.

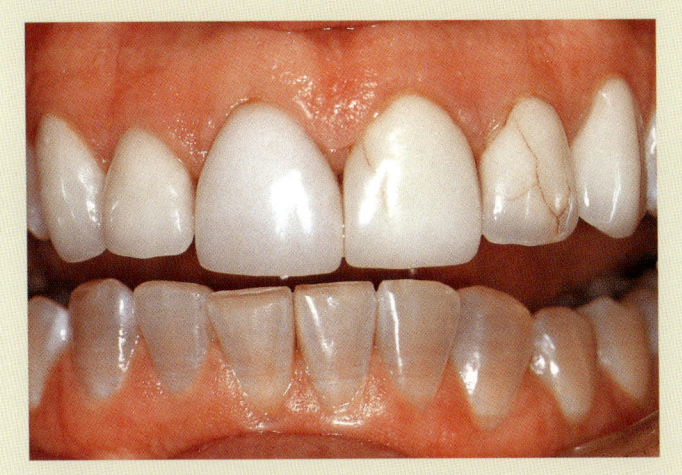

CASE 31　(80-81 page)
ポーセレンラミネートベニア(ノリタケAAA陶材使用)。
EX-3 Porcelain Laminate Veneer.

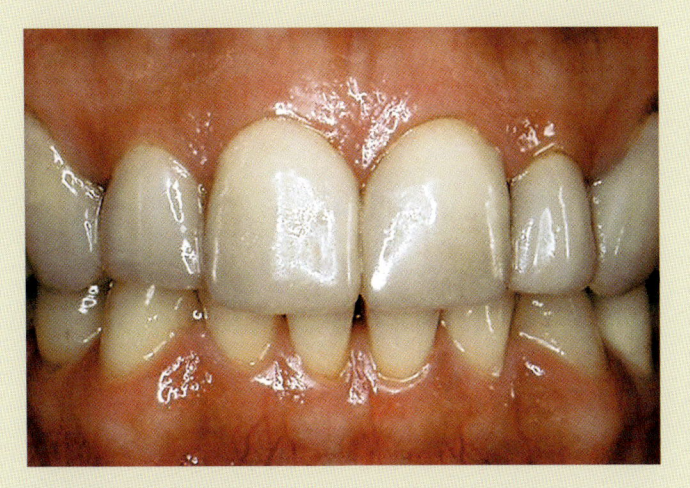

CASE 32　(82-83 page)
ポーセレンラミネートベニア(ノリタケAAA陶材使用)。
EX-3 Porcelain Laminate Veneer.

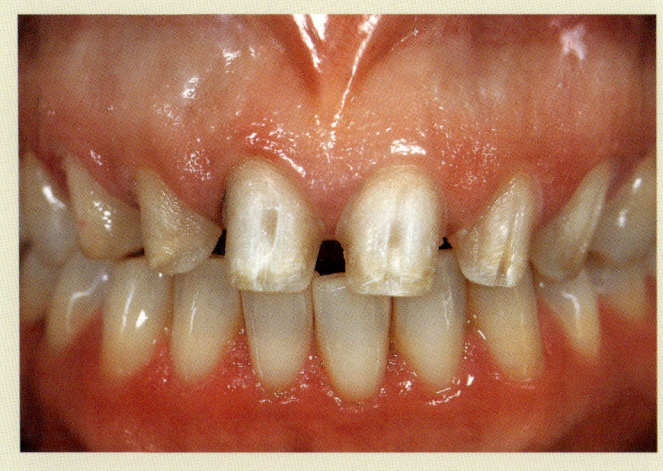

CASE 33　(84 page)
ポーセレンラミネートベニア(ノリタケAAA陶材使用)。
EX-3 Porcelain Laminate Veneer.

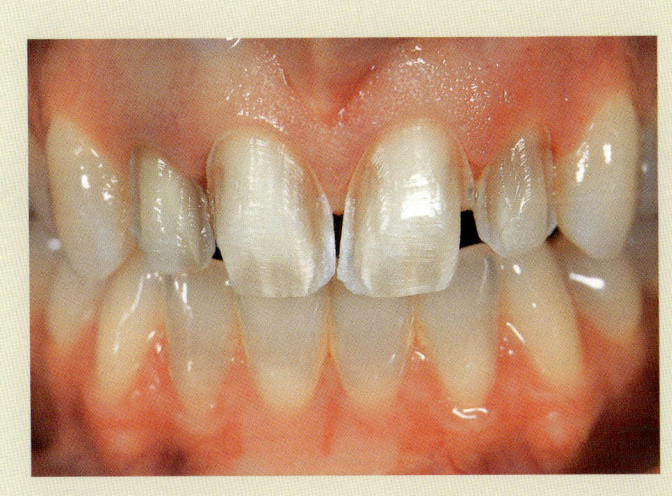

CASE 34　(85 page)
ポーセレンラミネートベニア(ノリタケAAA陶材使用)。
EX-3 Porcelain Laminate Veneer.

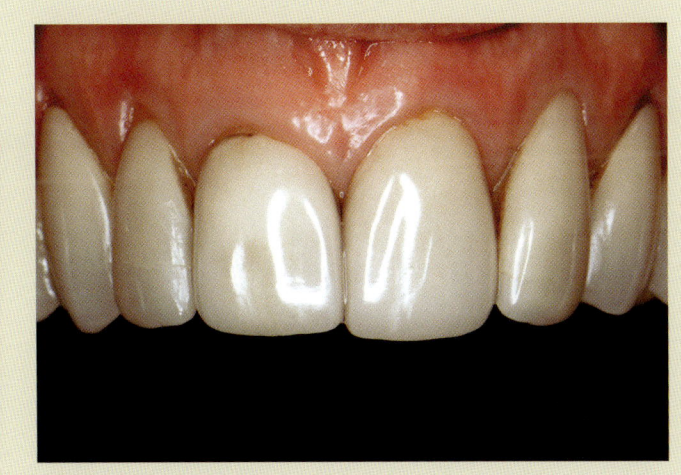

CASE 35　(86 page)
ポーセレンラミネートベニア(ノリタケAAA陶材使用)。
EX-3 Porcelain Laminate Veneer.

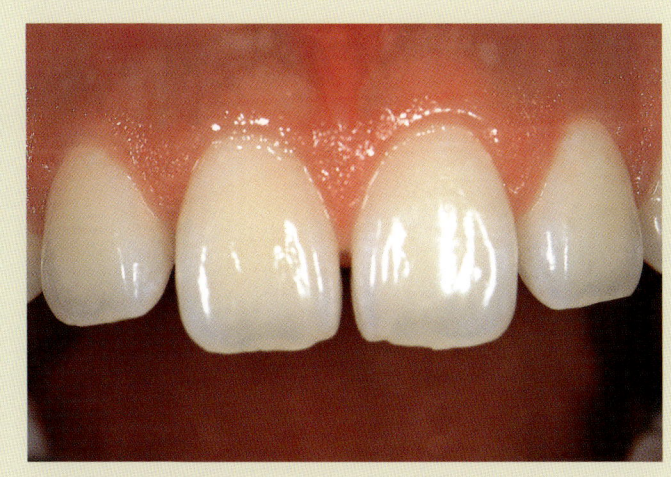

CASE 36　(87 page)
ポーセレンラミネートベニア(ノリタケAAA陶材使用)。
EX-3 Porcelain Laminate Veneer.

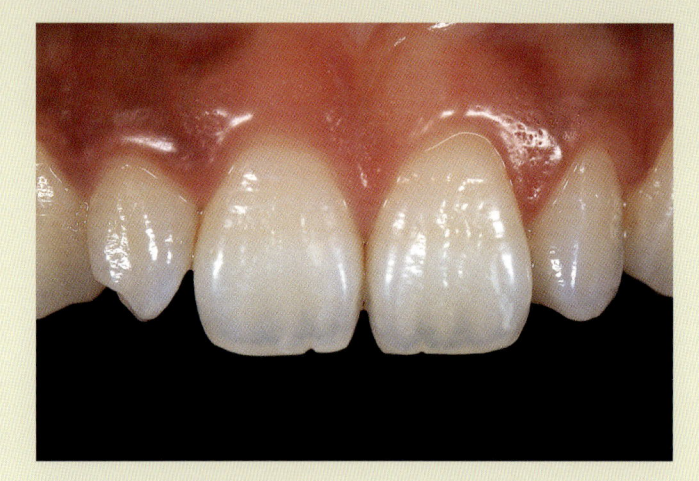

CASE 37 (88-89 page)
ポーセレンラミネートベニア(ノリタケAAA陶材使用)。
EX-3 Porcelain Laminate Veneer.

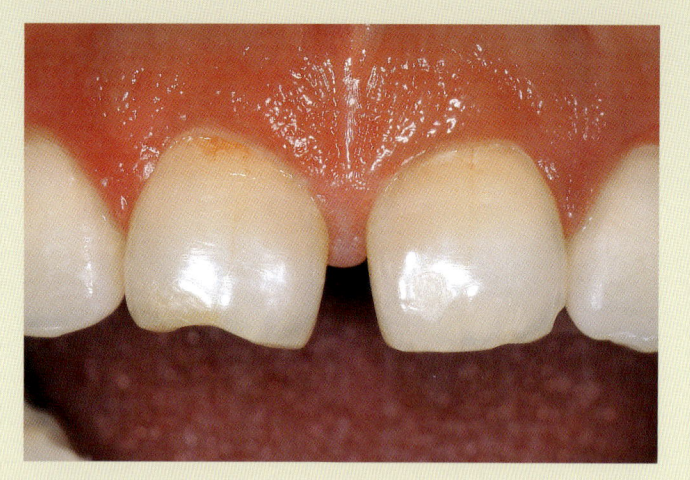

CASE 38 (90 page)
ポーセレンラミネートベニア(ノリタケAAA陶材使用)。
EX-3 Porcelain Laminate Veneer.

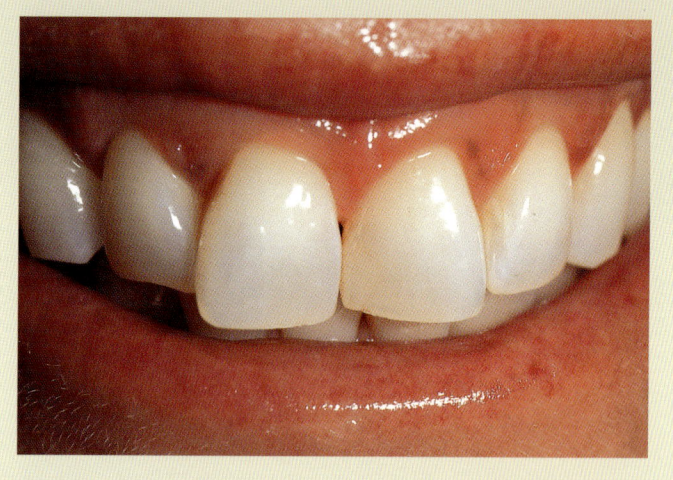

CASE 39 (91 page)
ポーセレンラミネートベニア(ノリタケAAA陶材使用)。
EX-3 Porcelain Laminate Veneer.

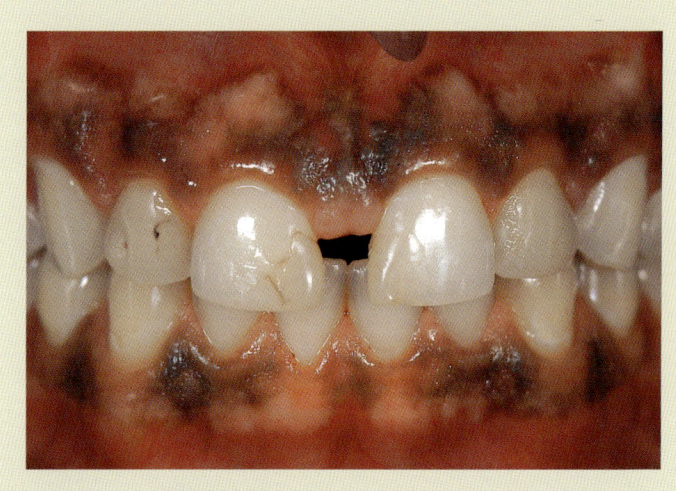

CASE 40 (92-93 page)
ポーセレンラミネートベニア(ノリタケAAA陶材使用)。
EX-3 Porcelain Laminate Veneer.

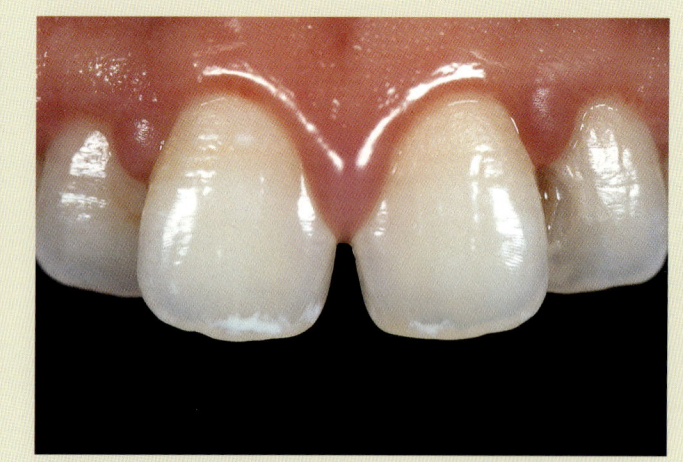

CASE 41 (94-95 page)
ポーセレンラミネートベニア(ノリタケAAA陶材使用)。
EX-3 Interproximal Porcelain Laminate Veneer.

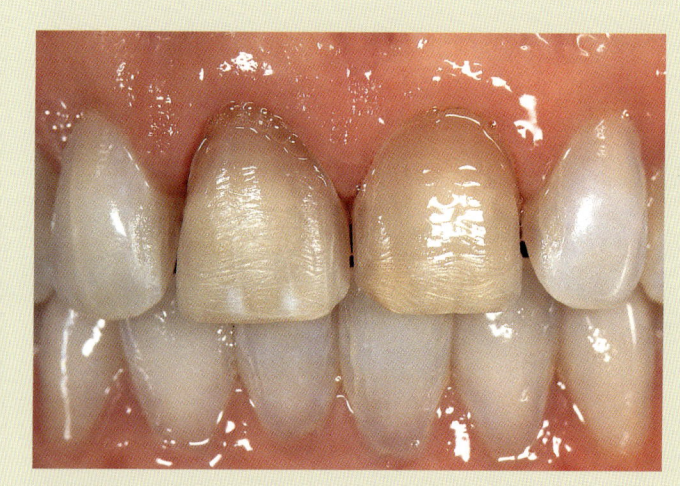

CASE 42 (96-97 page)
ポーセレンラミネートベニア(ノリタケAAA陶材使用)。
EX-3 Porcelain Laminate Veneer.

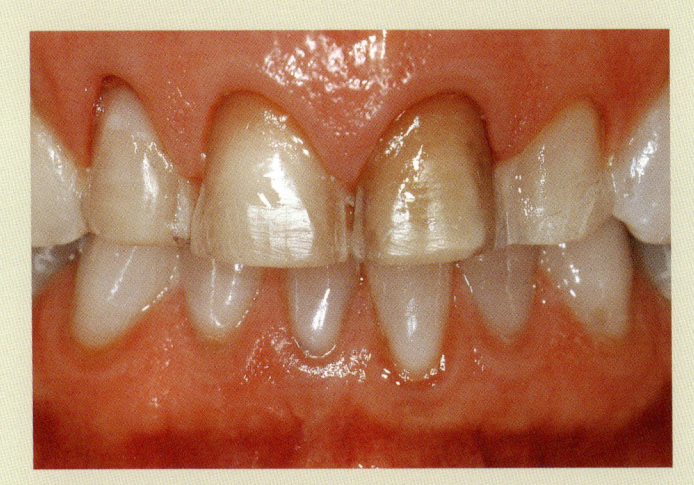

CASE 43 　(98 page)
ポーセレンラミネートベニア(ノリタケAAA陶材使用)。
EX-3 Porcelain Laminate Veneer.

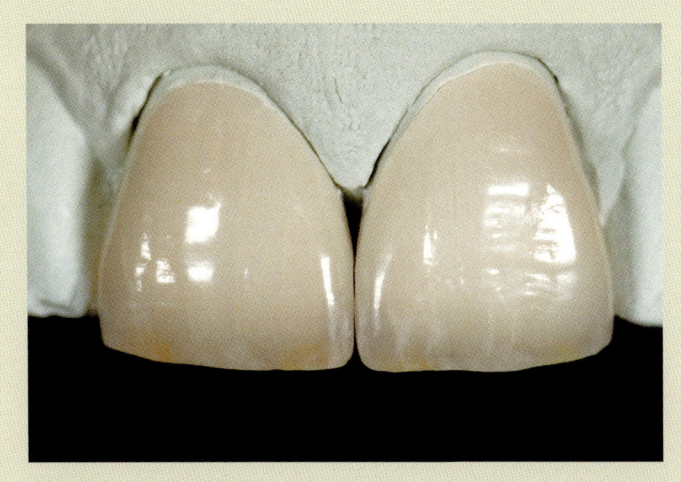

CASE 44 　(99 page)
ポーセレンラミネートベニア(ノリタケAAA陶材使用)。
EX-3 Porcelain Laminate Veneer.

Noritake
Noritake Dental Supply CO.,Limited

Nikon
株式会社 ニコン

* Art Womack D.D.S

* Christian W. Hahn D.D.S

* David J. Love D.D.S

* Hitoshi Aoshima R.D.T

* James E. Farthing D.D.S

* Kurt R. Schneider D.D.S

* Millard Roth D.D.S

* Phillip J. Martowski D.D.S

* Rodger K. Uchizono D.D.S

* Stuart R. Shlosberg D.D.S.,M.S.D

* Toshiro Yamada D.D.S

* Yuji Kayahara D.D.S

* Wayne Wu D.D.S

* William J. Capobianco D.D.S

Special Thanks

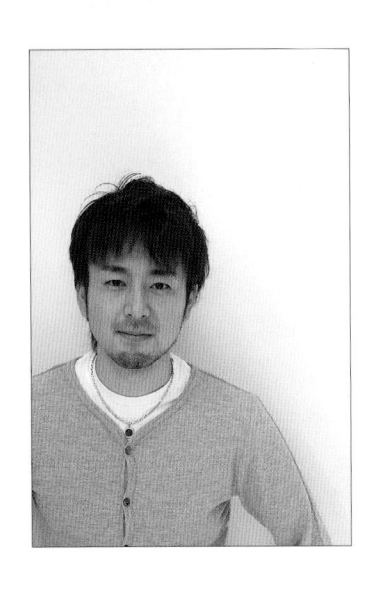

林　直樹（はやし　なおき）

プロフィール

1972年　東京都生まれ
1993年　大阪歯科大学附属歯科技工士専門学校卒業
1993年　株式会社　ナショナルデンタルラボラトリー入社
1999年　同社技術部主任　就任
2001年　同社退社
2001年　徳真会グループ　WORLD LAB U.S.A入社
2001年　早稲田歯科技工トレーニングセンター非常勤講師　就任
2002年　株式会社　ノリタケデンタルサプライ公認インストラクター認定
2003年　WORLD LAB U.S.Aを分社しUltimate Styles Dental Laboratory開設

A Diary　Through the Lens

2005年6月10日　第1版第1刷発行
2010年11月1日　第1版第2刷発行

著　者　　林　直樹

発 行 人　　佐々木一高

発 行 所　　クインテッセンス出版株式会社
　　　　　　東京都文京区本郷3丁目2番6号　〒113-0033
　　　　　　クイントハウスビル　電話　(03)5842-2270(代表)
　　　　　　　　　　　　　　　　　　　(03)5842-2272(営業部)
　　　　　　　　　　　　　　　　　　　(03)5842-2279(書籍編集部)
　　　　　　web page address　http://www.quint-j.co.jp/

印刷・製本　　サン美術印刷株式会社

Ⓒ2005　クインテッセンス出版株式会社　　禁無断転載・複写
Printed in Japan　　　　　　　落丁本・乱丁本はお取り替えします
　　　　　　　　　　ISBN978-4-87417-859-1　C3047

定価はケースに表示してあります